DE

To ......ions of
120 Homeopathic Remedies

J.H. Clarke

Arranged by
A. Gladstone Clarke

B. Jain Publishers (P) Ltd.
An ISO 9001 : 2000 Certified Company
USA—EUROPE—INDIA

DECACHORDS – TOP TEN INDICATIONS OF 120 HOMEOPATHIC REMEDIES

5th Impression: 2009

Published by Kuldeep Jain for
B. JAIN PUBLISHERS (P) LTD.
An ISO 9001 : 2000 Certified Company
1921/10, Chuna Mandi, Paharganj, New Delhi 110 055 (INDIA)
Tel.: 91-11-2358 0800, 2358 1100, 2358 1300, 2358 3100
Fax: 91-11-2358 0471 • *Email:* info@bjain.com
Website: **www.bjainbooks.com**

Printed in India by
Akash Press

ISBN: 978-81-319-0761-0

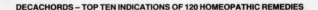

PUBLISHER'S NOTE

This new edition has been upgraded in the following ways:

- Abbreviations and names of drugs have been standardized according to *Synthesis* is the whole text.

- Improved and more readable font has been introduced with increased font size.

We hope all the above changes will make this new edition a pleasure to read.

Kuldeep Jain
MD, B. Jain Publishers

INTRODUCTION

This little effort arises from a felt need. It claims neither originality nor perfection. A suggestion made by Sir John Weir some years ago during a course of lectures to M.S.M. students led one of them to prepare for memorizing purposes a pocket note book giving in concise form the leading indications for about fifty remedies. Several students and missionary friends have since borrowed the book and profess to have found it helpful. It is now given this more permanent and extended form, though not without trepidation, in the sincere hope that others may be similarly benefited.

When first introduced to the materia medica the student is bewildered by the mass of symptoms presented under each drug and he often seeks in vain for a way out of the seeming maze. "Decachords" will provide the earnest student with some necessary clues guiding him to a practical acquaintance with the more frequently used remedies. The book is not a materia medica. Indications given are only the foundation upon which by further study and experience a fuller knowledge of homoeopathic drugs is to be built.

By request, a number of additional remedies have been included at the end of the book, the indications taking the form of "Pentachords". These bring the total of drugs dealt with up to one hundred and twenty, which may be considered a full *armamentum* for the missionary homoeopathist.

The notes are gathered from various sources. Due acknowledgements are made to Sir John Weir and Dr. Wheeler, whose valuable lectures have furnished much of the material.

Well-known works by Drs. Allen, Cowperthwaite, Nash and others have also been drawn upon for many keynotes.

On behalf of all who have taken the course at the Missionary School of Medicine the compiler takes this opportunity of expressing the deepest gratitude to past and present members of the teaching staff for their many patient and self-denying efforts. The labour has not been in vain. Former students now scattered in far distant lands as heralds of the gospel of Christ daily prove the healing art to be an invaluable aid in their work. They are also demonstrating beyond all doubt by many signal successes the truth of Hahnemann's dictum "Similia similibus curantur."

A.G.C.

Shantung, China.
December, 1925.

GENERAL HINTS

"Know your drugs by their peculiarities just as you recognize your friends not by the number of limbs but by their idiosyncrasies." (Dr. Margaret Tyler.)

Type and temperament do not rule out a remedy if other indications correspond. If present, however, they are a valuable confirmation.

Do not think that remedies particularly adapted to women are never indicated in the male sex. Sepia officinalis, for example, is frequently called for in men.

Never prescribe on one symptom alone but on the whole symptom-complex, remembering always that symptoms have a relative value. "Generals" and "mentals" rank first, then "peculiars" and finally "particulars." "Generals" are symptoms which the patient refers to his "ego," while "particulars" are referred to his complaint; e.g., "I feel worse in winter" is a general, but "My rheumatism is worse in cold weather" is a particular. "Particulars" are invariably emphasized by the patient.

As a rule unless symptoms are well marked they may be discarded.

Objective signs are usually of lower value than subjective symptoms except, perhaps, in straightforward acute diseases.

During the treatment of chronic cases old and often forgotten symptoms may make a temporary reappearance. These are not to be regarded as indications for a change of drug. When general improvement is being maintained minor incidental aches and pains may be ignored. Troublesome symptoms, however, sometimes call for an intercurrent remedy in a low potency.

Symptoms generally disappear curatively in the reverse order of their appearance.

It is seldom advisable to use a chronic remedy during the course of an acute ailment-choose the corresponding acute drug.

Golden rule. When definite improvement sets in, discontinue the administration of the remedy and do not repeat until the patient fails to show further reaction to the dose.

Continue with the same potency as long as it gives a reaction.

If the remedy be well chosen do not be in a hurry to change. In cases of apparent failure first try another potency (higher or lower) of the same drug.

When in doubt as to the advisiability of repeating or changing-wait!

High potencies often cause a preliminary aggravation.

Low potencies. 1x to 12x (6). Chiefly used in acute conditions and in frequent doses.

Medium potencies. 12 to 30. useful at the beginning of either acute of chronic cases, and especially when deep, organic changes are suspected.

High potencies. 200 up. Mostly used in chronic conditions and in infrequent doses.

Many drugs appear to be inert between 3x and 8x.

EXPLANATION OF SIGNS AND CONTRADICTIONS

< : The aggravation sign. > : The amelioration sign.

|| : Unaffected by.

Acc. by: Accompanied by.

Alt.: Alternating with.

Assoc.: Associated with.

Char.: Characteristic.

"Chilly": Predominantly < cold > warmth.

Ctr.: Contrast.

Esp.: Especially.

Gen.: Generally.

H/a: Headache.

M.P.: Menstrual period.

Rev.: Reverse.

T.B. Tuberculosis.

Temp.: Temporarily.

CONTENTS

Publisher's Note *(iii)*
Introduction *(v)*
General Hints *(vii)*
Explanation of Signs and Contradictions *(ix)*

Aconitum Napellus   1
Aesculus Hippocastanum   107
Agaricus Muscarius   2
Aloe Socotrina   108
Alumina   3
Ammonium Carbonicum   4
Anacardium Orientale   5
Antimonium Crudum   6
Antimonium Tartaricum   7
Apis Mellifica   8
Argentum Nitricum   9
Arnica Montana   10
Arsenicum Album   11
Aurum Metallicum   12
Baptisia Tinctoria   13
Baryta Carbonica   14
Belladonna   15
Benzoicum Acidum   109
Berberis Vulgaris   110
Bismuthum   111
Borax Veneta   16
Bromium   112

Bryonia Alba	17
Cactus Grandiflorus	113
Calcarea Phosphorica	20
Calcera Carbonica	18
Calendula Officinalis	114
Camphora Officinalis	21
Cantharivesicatoria	22
Capsicum Annuum	115
Carbo Animalis	116
Carbo Vegetabilis	23
Caulophyllum Thalictroides	117
Causticum	24
Chamomilla	26
Chelidonium Majus	28
Cicuta Virosa	118
Cimicifugaracemosa	29
Cina Maritima	119
Cinchona Officinalis	31
Cocculus Indicus	32
Coffea Cruda	33
Colchicum Autumnale	34
Colocynthis	120
Conium Maculatum	35
Crocus Sativus	121
Crotalus Horridus	122
Cuprum Metallicum	36
Digitalis Purpurea	123
Drosera Rotundifolia	124
Dulcamara	125
Eupatorium Perfoliatum	126
Euphrasia Officinalis	127
Ferrum Metallicum	37

Ferrum Phosphoricum   128
Fluoricum Acidum   129
Gelsemium Sempervirens   39
Glonoinum   130
Graphites   41
Hamamelis Virginiana   131
Helleborus Niger   132
Hepar Sulphur   42
Hyoscyamus Niger   133
Hypericum Perforatum   134
Ignatia Amara   44
Iodium   46
Ipecacuanha   47
Kalium Bichromicum   48
Kalium Bromatum   135
Kalium Carbonicum   49
Kalmia Latifolia   136
Kreosotum   51
Lac Caninum   52
Lachesis Mutus   53
Ledumpalustre   55
Lilium Tigrinum   57
Lycopodium Clavatum   58
Magnesium Carbonicum   60
Magnesium Phosphoricum   137
Medorrhinum   61
Mercurius (Vivus or Solubilis)   62
Mercurius Corrosivus   138
Mezereum   64
Muriaticum Acidum   139
Natrium Carbonicum   65
Natrium Muriaticum   66
Natrium Sulphuricum   68

Nitricum Acidum	69
Nux Moschata	70
Nux Vomica	71
Opium	73
Petroleum	74
Phosphoricum Acidum	75
Phosphorus	76
Phytolacca Decandra	78
Platina	79
Plumbum Metallicum	80
Podophyllum Peltatum	81
Psorinum	82
Pulsatilla Nigricans	83
Pyrogenium	140
Ranunculus Bulbosus	141
Rhus Toxicodendron	85
Ruta Graveolens	142
Sanguinaria Canadensis	87
Secale Cornutum	88
Sepia Officinalis	89
Silicea Terra	91
Spigelia Anthelmia	143
Spongia Tosta	144
Stannum Metallicum	145
Staphysagria	93
Stramonium	146
Sulphur	95
Syphilinum	97
Thuja Occidentalis	98
Tuberculinum	100
Veratrum Album	102
Veratrum Viride	104
Zincum Metallicum	105

ACONITUM NAPELLUS

1. Strong, healthy, full-blooded person of quick, lively, sanguine temperament.

2. Emotional, mental and physical **tension**; hyperæsthesia, of the special senses.

3. **Onset of sthenic fevers,** characterized by (a) **intense anxiety** with prediction and **fear of death,** causing **restlessness** and tossing about; (b) strong, full, rapid pulse; (c) **dry, hot skin** and great thirst; (d) intolerance of warmth, bed clothes thrown off.

4. Complaints from exposure to **dry, cold winds** and draughts, also from suppressed perspiration, mental emotions (esp. fright), injury, shock, surgical operation, intense heat.

5. Pains intense and insupportable; tearing, stabbing, cutting.

6. Pains often associated with local numbness or tingling.

7. Sudden disturbances of the special sense, esp. vision.

8. Sudden spasmodic affections in children, esp. **croup.**

9. Haemorrhages of bright-red blood when the characteristic mental anxiety is present.

10. **Modalities;** < evening and night; warm room, lying on left side; > fresh air; joint pain < motion > rest.

Notes : Chronic–**Sulphur,** Keynote–**Tension.**

AGARICUS MUSCARIUS

1. Light-haired persons of lax fibre; old people with weak circulation; drunkards.

2. Deliriums; in typhoid conditions; of silly kind; constant raving, tries to get out of bed (occupies position between Stram. and Lach.); delirium tremens.

3. **Burning, itching and redness** of various parts which are swollen and hot; **chilblains, frostbite,** etc. (locally and internally).

4. Spasmodic conditions; tremors, twitchings; involuntary movements while awake, cease when asleep; **choreas,** from jerking of single muscles to dancing of whole body.

5. Spine sensitive to touch; painful at every turn of the body; backache < while sitting.

6. Headaches; esp. in drunkards after debauch; or from prolonged desk work.

7. Asthenia from prolonged strain spasm of accommodation; twitching of eyes and lids; weakness of muscles; swimming of type; myopia; chronic choroiditis.

8. Irritable heart of tea and coffee drinkers and tobacco smokers; irregular, tumultuous palpitation.

9. Symptoms appear diagonally; upper left and lower right (Led.; ctr. Med.).

10. **Modalities;** < cold air; damp; before thunder.

ALUMINA

1. Dark, spare withered-looking subjects; disposition gen. mild and cheerful.

2. Attacks of depression. Loss of memory; time passes slowly.

3. Great dryness of all mucous membranes (except female genitalia) with sense of constriction.

4. Abnormal appetite, craving for indigestible things; potatoes disagree.

5. **Inactivity of the rectum**; no desire and no ability until large accumulation, even **soft stool requires great straining**; stool hard and knotty or soft, clayey and adhesive.

6. **Leucorrhoea, acrid**, transparent, **profuse, running down to the heels** (Syph.) < daytime; gen, assoc. delayed, scanty menses after which patient physically and mentally exhausted.

7. Paralytic weakness of **lower limbs** with great heaviness and **lack of co-ordination**; "must sit down"; also with burning pain esp. in the back.

8. Chronic throat conditions, "every cold settles in the throat."

9. Skin eruptions < winter; intolerable itching < warmth of bed; < starchy foods and all irritating things (salt, pepper, etc.).

10. **Modalities.** Patient chilly < cold except headache; at new and full moon; on alternate days; > eating.

Notes : A chornic of **Bryonia alba**. Slow but long-acting chronic remedy.

AMMONIUM CARBONICUM

1. Stout, fleshy persons of sedentary habit; delicate women who faint easily and fly to smelling bottle on least excuse; old people.

2. Listlessness; ill-humour esp. during stormy weather; desire for olfactory stimulants.

3. Hæmorrhagic diathesis; **epistaxis, when washing face**, after eating; venous congestions.

4. Tendency to gangrenous degeneration of parts; whole body seems overpowered by toxic effects of the disease (Ail., Bapt.).

5. Affections of respiratory tract; acute and chronic; **stoppage of nose mostly at night**, must breathe through mouth (a keynote even in diptheria); catarrha, coryzas; chronic bronchitis esp. of the aged and when associated with emphysema; asthma, coughs, etc., gen. < 3-4 a.m.

6. Malignant scarlatina with somnolence; threatened paralysis of brain; toxic effects appear to center in the throat, which is dark red, putrid, externally swollen.

7. All discharges acrid, excoriating, leaving rawness and burning.

8. **Cholera-like symptoms at commencement of M.P.**; menses premature, profuse with great fatigue and < of all symptoms.

9. Affections mostly right-sided.

10. **Modalities**; < cold, wet weather; washing; during M.P.

Note : Useful locally for stings of insects, etc.

ANACARDIUM ORIENTALE

1. Persons of sedentary habits suffering from brain-fag; nervous, hysterical women esp. during pregnancy.

2. Mentals: Patients distressed by **sudden loss of memory**; lacks self-confidence; fears inability to "get through" (Arg-n., Lyc.); paradoxical temper-laughs at serious matters, serious over laughable things; great suspicion. Dual personality, as of **two wills acting in opposition. Irresistible desire to curse and swear** (Lac-c., Lil-t., Nit-a.).

3. Weakness of all the senses.

4. Neuralgic pains, dull, penetrating or pressing as from a blunt instrument or plug.

5. Sense of constriction as of a hoop round the part (Cact.).

6. Gastric symptoms > while eating.

7. Ineffectual urging to stool.

8. Complaints prone to go from right to left.

9. Skin eruptions with excessive itching, similar to Rhus-t.

10. Patient generally chilly; < damp; mental exertion; all symptoms > **while eating except cough.**

ANTIMONIUM CRUDUM

1. Adapted to the extremes of life; esp. to young people inclined to grow fat.

2. Mentals: **Great sadness** with weeping, esp. in intermittents. Sulkness, no wish to speak to people. In women, sentimental mood even ecstatic love, in the moonlight.

3. In **children**, fretful, peevish disposition; temper at every little attention; **cannot bear to be touched.**

4. Gastric disorders esp. from overeating; **thick, milky-white coated tongue**; loathing of food, nausea and tendency to vomit; desire for acids which <.

5. Crusts and cracks about the nostrils and labial commissures.

6. Corns and callosities esp. on the soles of the feet-very tender when walking; deformed nails.

7. Alternation of constipation and watery diarrhoea esp. in old people.

8. Torpid state of the mucous membranes with excessive secretion; esp. mucous piles, continual oozing discharge staining yellow.

9. Reappearing symptoms change locality.

10. **Modalities**; < extremes of cold and heat; from taking cold esp. cold bathing; sun heat and radiated heat though many symptoms are > by heat.

ANTIMONIUM TARTARICUM

1. Phlegmatic subjects; hydrogenoid constitutions.

2. Persistent, irreconcible **ill-humour**, < consolation; child fractious, complaining, resents least touch (Ant-c.).

3. Respiratory troubles with **great accumulation of mucus**; coarse rales; no explusive power yet if expectorates temporarily >; attacks of suffocative dyspnoea with **cyanosis**.

4. Prostration with great **drowsiness** and cold sweat.

5. Gastric troubles with nausea and vomiting; latter temp. > (rev. lp.); loathing of food; moist, heavily coated white tongue; desire for acids (esp. apples) which <; < milk.

6. Choleraic diarrhoea; stools slimy, generally yellow or brown, occasionally bloody.

7. Fever with shiverings and marked sense of cold; violent but short-lasting sensations of heat; pulse rapid and weak; sweat profuse and exhausting; thirst for cold water little and often. (Ars.).

8. Violent pain in sacro-lumbar region; slightest movement causes vomiting and cold sweat.

9. Widespread pustular eruptions. Small-pox (Variolinum).

10. **Modalities**; < heat and < cold, damp weather evening towards night; anger or vexation.

APIS MELLIFICA

1. Strumous constitutions; children and girls who become awkward esp. in handling things; hysterical women.

2. Anxiety with tearful restlessness; impaired memory and absent-mindedness in elderly persons.

3. **Oedematous swellings**, serous effusions, and urticaria.

4. **Pains burning, darting, stinging** > cold (rev. Ars.).

5. General soreness and sensitiveness of body surface < touch or pressure esp. uterine and ovarian regions; constriction disliked; weary, bruised feeling.

6. Marked **restlessness** (physical causes) without > to symptoms.

7. Great drowsiness; sleep much disturbed by pain or anxious dreams; sopor interrupted by piercing screams (meningitis).

8. **Thirstlessness** in nearly all complaints esp. dropsical conditions.

9. Ailments right-sided or travel from right to left.

10. Patients < **all forms of heat**; general < 4-6 p.m. < sleep.

Notes : Slow-acting remedy. In acute conditions wait an hour or two. Low potencies should not be given during pregnancy. Keynote.–**Oedema**.

ARGENTUM NITRICUM

1. Subjects withered, old-looking through disease, esp. after unusual or, long-continued mental exertion; children.

2. Hypochondriasis; **lacks self-confidence**; apprehensive, hurried, discontented, time passes slowly; suicidal impulses.

3. General debility with nervous tremors.

4. Strange sensations; (a) of expansion in various parts, (b) as of splinter, esp. in the throat, (c) as if objects project towards the patient.

5. Catarrhal conditions of the mucous membranes; profuse, muco-purulent discharges (Puls.) and ulceration.

6. Gastric ailments with much flatulence and **violent, difficult belchings**; < food; great **craving for sweets** which <.

7. Diarrhoeas; **psychic** (Gels.); catarrhal, spluttering, grass-green, < drinking, sweets; also dysentery, advanced cases.

8. Spinal complaints; sensitiveness of the spine; defective co-ordination of muscles esp. of lower limbs; lightning-like pains; epileptiform convulsions; paralysis.

9. Metrorrhagia with nervous erythism at climaxis.

10. Patient < heat, must have fresh air yet chilly when uncovered; < **mental exertion**; at M.P.; pains esp. h/a < dancing > tight pressure; backache > standing.

ARNICA MONTANA

1. Acts best in sanguine, plethoric subjects.

2. Oversensitiveness to pain; great **fear of being touched** or struck by anyone coming near, esp. in gout and rheumatic conditions.

3. **Bruised, sore feeling all over; bed feels too hard** (Bapt.).

4. **Injuries** esp. to soft parts; **bruises** (Ham.); strains (Rhus-t.); concussions (Hyper.); results of injuries however remote; hæmorrhages esp. of mechanical origin.

5. Typhoid states; indifference or stupor; answers questions correctly but unconsciousness immediately returns; involuntary stool and urine or long interval between stools.

6. Discharges offensive; eructations, flatus, etc., have odours as of "rotten eggs."

7. Head hot, body cold; or heat of upper part of body; also deathly coldness of forearm in children.

8. Tendency to small, painful boils one succeeding another.

9. Prevents suppuration and septicæmia; excellent after parturition esp. if instrumental delivery.

10. **Modalities**; < rest; lying down; > motion.

Keynote : **Trauma.**

ARSENICUM ALBUM

1. Fat, plethoric persons; usually dark; easy disposition to diarrhoea, vegetarians; old people.

2. Combination of sadness and irritability; sometimes suicidal tendency; great **fastidiousness**; fear of the dark; < alone; hyperæthesia of the special senses.

3. In adynamic fevers; rapid and **great prostration yet marked restlessness from anxiety and fear of death** (Acon.); wants to be moved from place to place; obviously ill and lacking in vital power. Septic states.

4. **Burning**, lancinating **pains** and sensations > **heat** (rev. Phos.).

5. **Discharges burning**, excorating offensive, debilitating, thin, watery; generally scanty.

6. **Periodicity** and **malignancy** of symptoms.

7. Great **thirst**; calls **for small quantities at frequent intervals.**

8. Gastric ailments with loathing of food; vomits everything even a spoonful of water; ill-effects of eating fruit, ices, etc., also ptomaine and similar poisonings. Patient dislikes meat but desires fat.

9. Skin troubles of all kinds, esp. scaly eruptions.

10. Patient very chilly, < cold and damp; lying with head low; **midnight to 3 a.m.**; rest: > heat, except head symptoms.

Note : Thuj. is sometimes its chronic.

AURUM METALLICUM

1. Sanguine, ruddy persons with dark hair and eyes; old people; scrofulous or mercurio-syphilitic subjects.

2. **Profound melancholia** with desire for death and **suicidal** tendencies; often connected with liver troubles in men; with uterine troubles in women.

3. Specially adapted to **pining boys**, low-spirited, lifeless, lacking vim; testes undeveloped.

4. Hypersensitiveness; to contradiction, to pain; of the special senses.

5. Ailments resulting from strong mental emotions.

6. Intense, deep seated boring pains < night.

7. **Caries of bones**, esp. nasal, palatine and mastoid, with deep ulceration and horribly offensive discharges.

8. Interstitial changes in various organs, esp. heart, liver and kidneys.

9. Hemiopia; sees only lower half of objects.

10. **Modalities**; < cold, damp weather; **sunset to sunrise**; warmth of bed; at M.P.

BAPTISIA TINCTORIA

1. Low septic fevers with great prostration and muttering delirium; face dark red; vacant, stupid, even besotted expression.

2. Great **mental confusion**; sensation of divided personality expressed in various ways, e.g., body feels scattered, tries to collect the pieces. Concentration difficult (falls asleep while being spoken to or while answering question).

3. Numbness and soreness; aching, **bruised, sore feeling all over; bed feels too hard** (Arn.).

4. Putrescence of all discharges, secretions and exhalations.

5. Absence of acute pain.

6. Drowsiness and languor; restless sleep.

7. Mouth and tongue very dry in fevers; tongue at first white with red papillæ and red edges; later, yellow-brown center, edges dark red and shining; then brown, parched, cracked and ulcerated; sordes.

8. Frequent, loose, dark, acrid, offensive, debilitating stools (Ars.).

9. Ulceration of mucous membranes esp. of fauces; with dark-red appearance, absence of pain; can swallow only liquids.

10. No marked reaction to temperature though gen. some < cold; gen. < movement; on waking.

Note : An acute and sub-acute remedy.

BARYTA CARBONICA

1. Dwarfish, ill-nourished children or childish old people; scrofulous subjects esp. when fat.

2. **Mental** and bodily; **weakness**; semi-imbecility.

3. Great tendency to glandular swellings and indurations, esp. of **tonsils**, acute and chronic; also fatty tumours.

4. Patient easily catches cold, esp. in the throat; subject to quinsy.

5. Paralysis and other affections arising from impaired brain function.

6. Degenerative changes in walls of arteries. Atheroma, etc.

7. Diseases peculiar to old men. Prostatic troubles, etc.

8. Offensive foot sweats and ailments (esp. of throat) following suppression; one-sided sweats.

9. Left side mostly affected.

10. **Modalities**; < cold, damp; washing affected parts, < when thinking of his disease.

BELLADONNA

1. Plethoric persons inclined to obesity and subject to sudden congestions of the head; happy when well, violent when sick.

2. **Brain symptoms predominate**; (a) wild delirium; fantastic illusions or rage with destructive mania; (b) constant moaning, starting or jumping in or on going to sleep, even to springing out of bed.

3. Hyperæsthesia of all the senses; every stimulus almost intolerable.

4. Acute local inflammations with **sudden onset** and rapid course, before products have formed; esp. of peritoneum.

5. Fevers with dry, burning hot skin, sweat only on covered parts, smooth, shiny, scarlet surface; **flushed face**, sparkling eyes with dialted pupils, **throbbing carotids**; pulse rapid and full but not tense.

6. Severe, paroxysmal pains of various kinds but gen. **throbbing**; sudden onset, indefinite course, sudden decline, often < lying down (except joint pains), < heat.

7. Dryness of mucous membranes esp. of throat.

8. Great bearing down in the female organs; menses premature and profuse, flow bright red and hot.

9. Ailments predominantly right-sided.

10. Patients chilly, < cold but < heat of sun; < night or 3 p.m. to 3 a.m.; every stimulus, least jar of bed > wrapping up, warmth; resting in semi-recumbent position; lying on unaffected side.

Notes : Chronic–Calc. Action swift but not very prolonged. Suitable for acute and sub-acute condition. Do not give low potencies to nursing mothers.

BORAX VENETA

1. Children at dentition period; young women.

2. Excessive nervousness; slightest sudden noise frightens.

3. **Great dread of downward motion** in nearly all complaints; child clings to nurse and cries when it is being put down.

4. **Aphthous ulcerations** of mucous membranes; of mouth with heat, tenderness, great thirst, etc., prevents child from nursing; from dental plate in old people; ulcers bleed easily, < **touch, eating** salty or sour food; often assoc. diarrhoea of yellow or green stools day and night.

5. Functional urinary troubles in children; urine frequent; scanty, hot, with burning, shooting pains causing child to scream before passing (Lyc., Sanic., Sars.).

6. Profuse, albuminous, **leucorrhoea** with sensation as of warm water flowing down; erosions of os and cervix (internally and locally).

7. Unhealthy skin; every injury suppurates; nostrils crusty, inflamed; tip of nose shining red. In young women hair becomes frowsy and tangled, splits; ingrowing eyelashes, etc.

8. Stitching pains in various localities esp. right chest on deep inspiration or coughing.

9. Wakes early a.m. and cannot fall asleep again for two hours owing to heat in whole body esp. head; child screams out in sleep as if frightened by dreams.

10. **Modalities**; < damp, cold weather; pains usually > pressure.

BRYONIA ALBA

1. Dark persons of firm, fleshy fibre; choleric temperament; bilious and rheumatic tendencies.

2. Fever. Patient lies like a log, < least movement, resents any interference or questioning; at night, active delirium or broken sleep; disturbed about immediately personal concerns; vague, inconstant desires; wants to go home (Cimic., Hyos.).

3. Inflammatory affections of serous membranes; when effusion is about to occur; also **mastitis**, mammæ heavy, hard, hot, pale.

4. Sharp, **stitching pains** (Kali–C.) < **motion**, > rest.

5. Excessive **dryness** of all mucous membranes from lips to rectum (resulting, e.g., in 6 and 7); secretions scanty.

6. **Great thirst** for copious draughts at long intervals (rev. Ars.).

7. Constipation; stools large, hard, dark, dry, crumbling as if burnt; also summer diarrhoeas from chill or overheating.

8. Gastric disorders; foul, yellow-coated tongue; capricious appetite; sensation as of stone in stomach (Nux–v., Puls.).

9. Ailments chiefly right-sided (ovarian troubles often an exception).

10. **Modalities**; < **slightest motion of any kind**; at night esp. about 9 p.m. or early a.m. even after good sleep; < heat, esp. sun heat; > **absolute rest**, mental and physical; cool air and applications; lying on painful side.

Notes : Chronic remedies, Nat– m., Alum., Lyc.. Useful in ailments from suppression of discharges and acute exanthema.

CALCERA CARBONICA

1. Lecophlegmatic subjects; "fair, fat, flabby"; **children** with tendency to **grow fat**; large head and abdomen; slow development of mind and body; slow and imperfect ossification (difficult, delayed dentition, open fontanelles, etc.). Girls who **grow too rapidly**.

2. Anxiety of mind; all kinds of nervous apprehension with difficulty expressed and combated; fears insanity; night terrors; children **slow** to learn though often painstaking and industrious.

3. **Easy sweating**; of single parts; **of the head, wetting pillow far around when asleep**.

4. Deficient circulation; **coldness** of single parts; cold, clammy feeling esp. of legs and feet, also hands.

5. General sourness esp. of alimentary system.

6. Digestion weak with much fermentation; craving for eggs esp. during illness; for indigestible things; constipation the rule, pale, clayey stools; dentition diarrhoeas. Sinking sensations in abdomen (any time).

7. Menses premature, profuse, protracted; < least mental excitement; profuse leucorrhoea between periods.

8. Conditions arising from loss of body fluids (Chin; Ph–A.) esp. nervous symptoms.

9. Chronic glandular enlargement and unhealthy skin; itching eruptions, warts, small non-malignant growths, rhagades.

10. Patient very chilly; < cold and damp; from working in water; 2 to 3 a.m.; > warmth yet on getting warm is overwarm; gen. > when constipated; > lying painful side.

Notes : This remedy is slow in developing its action. Chronic of Belladonna. Keynote–Slow Development.

CALCAREA PHOSPHORICA

1. Thin, spare subjects with dark complexion and **inclined to emaciate**. Scrofulous, rachitic children during first and especially second dentition. (Heads sweats not so prominent a symptom as in Calc. and Sil.). Girls at or near puberty.

2. **Sunken, flabby abdomen** in children with general emaciation and inability to stand.

3. Gastro-intestinal disorders < at every attempt to eat, vomiting of undigested food esp. milk; craving for salt or smoked meats.

4. Dentition diarrhoeas; green stools with offensive flatus.

5. Patient **feels complaints more when thinking about them**. (Helon., Ox–ac.).

6. Other general indications similar to Calc.

7. Chronic catarrhal conditions with tendency to polypi and overgrowth of lymphatic tissue.

8. Non-union of fractures esp. in old people; promotes formation of callus.

9. Debility remaining after acute diseases esp. in young people.

10. **Modalities;** < cold and damp, particularly from **melting snows** (in rheumatic complaints, etc.); < spring and autumn; > after lying down.

CAMPHORA OFFICINALIS

1. Scrofulous children are most sensitive to this remedy; blonde type.

2. Great præcordial anxiety and restlessness.

3. **Sudden and complete prostration** of the vital forces; hippocratic face, husky voice, etc., even after surgical operations.

4. **Body surface cold** yet patient does not feel cold and **cannot bear covering** (with less suddenness-Sec.).

5. Initial stages of **cholera**, colds, etc. before discharges are established.

6. Colic, cramps and convulsions with mental anguish.

7. Pains disappear when thinking of them (rev. Calc–p., etc.).

8. Sudden retrocession of eruptions or suppression of discharges.

9. Antidotes most vegetable poisons including tobacco, mushrooms, etc.

10. Complaints > open air; profuse sweat.

Notes : Best administered as Rubini's tincture on sugar. Keynote–**Collapse**. Advisable to keep this drug away from all others owing to its antidotal action.

CANTHARIVESICATORIA

1. In acute diseases with **intense irritation** both mental and physical.

2. Mental irritability, < by the pains; paroxysms of passion.

3. Genito-urinary disorders with **constant urging** and the characteristic pains before, during and after micturition (Cann–s.); urine passes only in drops; < drinking.

4. **Violent cutting, burning pains** with spasms; sore, raw, burning sensations.

5. Intense inflammations of the skin with the formation of vesicles.

6. Violent inflammations of serous membranes with effusion and the characteristic pains.

7. Hæmorrhages from mucous orifices.

8. Violent erythism of the sexual organs.

9. Burns and scalds before or just after blisters form. (Externally and internally, well diluted.)

10. **Modalities**; < touch; drinking; > warmth.

CARBO VEGETABILIS

1. Cachetic, venous, sluggish, even stupid, old people. Persons whose vitality is weakened by exhausting diseases, loss of body fluids, or injuries.

2. Mental torpor; memory weak; indolence; fear of the dark.

3. Extreme prostration; **last stages** in any disease with hippocratic face; blueness; cold feet and legs to knees; cold sweat breath, etc.; thready intermittent pulse.

4. Alimentary disorders with much fermentation; **excessive accumulation of gas** < upper part of abdomen; < lying down; > passing wind up or down; plainest food disagrees; dislikes meat esp. fat, fat foods (Puls.) even milk.

5. Very offensive discharges.

6. Burning sensations or pains in various organs.

7. Venous, passive, persistent hæmorrhages from any mucous outlet.

8. Spasmodic respiratory complaints esp. in the aged; < cold air after warm room; discharge yellow, profuse. Hoarseness and aphonia < evenings and damp air.

9. Lack of reaction to well-selected remedies.

10. Patient chilly yet must have air; **"wants to be fanned"** (Chin.); < overheating; at M.P.; constriction.

CAUSTICUM

1. Dark-haired persons of rigid fibre and yellow, sallow complexion.

2. Melancholy mood; esp. after long-lasting grief or sorrow; with easy weeping particularly in children; or peevishness and pessimism; no disposition or ability for physical and mental exertion; intense sympathy for the sufferings of others.

3. Faint-like sinking of strength with internal trembling (Gels.).

4. **Paralytic conditions of single parts**; gen. **right-sided**; of rectum, resulting in constipation with constant ineffectual desire and tendency to stand during stool; also gradually appearing general paralysis.

5. Rheumatic affections with feeling of tension and shortening of muscles; tearing, drawing pains; more in limbs than in joints.

6. Great **rawness and soreness** in various parts; some times described as burning.

7. Cough, hollow, spasmodic; often with **hoarseness** or aphonia; < on expiration, > cold drink; acc. by spurt of urine; tough stringy mucus difficult to expectorate.

8. Unhealthy skin; great tendency to warts; ailments from suppressed chronic skin troubles.

9. Great restlessness at night; unable to find easy position to lie in.

10. Patient chilly; < in clear, fine weather, > damp, wet weather (i.e., mild, soft air) yet < from bathing or getting wet.

Note : Incompatible with Phosphorus; must not be used before or after.

CHAMOMILLA

1. Adapted to nervous, excitable temperaments, esp. in women and children; children during dentition; rheumatic diathesis.

2. Every degree of ill-temper; fits of **spiteful irritability**; uncivil even to best friends (no underlying ill nature like Nux–v.); confesses the fault but repeats it; affirms "cannot help it, I feel so." **Children** peevish, nothing pleases, **quiet only when carried** and petted.

3. **Oversensitiveness** to all unpleasant stimuli esp. **pain** which **seems intolerable**, at night causing patient to jump out of bed and walk about, pain acc. by and alt. with numbness.

4. Great sense of debility out of all proportions to the seriousness of the disease.

5. All discharges hot (sweat, stools, etc.).

6. Local heat; of hands and feet, **one cheek flushed** and hot, the other pale and cold.

7. Dentition diarrhoeas; hot, acrid, green stools; odour of rotten eggs.

8. Menstrual and puerperal disorders with char. pains and irritability; menses excessive with dark clots.

9. Aliments from anger and violent excitement; also from abuse of stimulants.

10. Patient < heat and hot applications yet not > by cold; sensitive to damp, cold weather and to **high winds** esp. about the ears; < evening and night.

Note : A swift-acting but not very searching remedy.
Keynote : **Oversensitiveness.**

CHELIDONIUM MAJUS

1. Thin, fair-complexioned subjects tendency to gastric and hepatic complaints.

2. Hypochondriasis with lethargy; drowsiness and debility.

3. **Constant pain under the lower angle of right shoulder blade.**

4. Hepatic diseases with or without the char. pain; soreness, swelling and pain in liver region; tongue coated yellow with red margin showing imprint of teeth (sometimes white-coated); diarrhoea of yellow or clay-coloured stools; skin and sclerotics jaundiced.

5. Gastric disorders with nausea; desire for and > from very hot drinks; > taking food; aversion from cheese.

6. Neuralgias esp. of head and face with profuse lachrymation from the right eye.

7. Rheumatic complaints; joints swollen, hot, stiff and tender; > hot applications.

8. Respiratory troubles esp. with hepatic complications; cough loose, rattling but expectoration difficult; oppressed breathing; larynx feels as if full of dust.

9. Markedly affects the **right side**; very seldom indicated in left-sided complaints.

10. Patient gen. < heat yet most symptoms > heat; < towards evening (Lyc.); < movement; > eating.

CIMICIFUGARACEMOSA

(Actæa Racemosa)

1. Thin, single women with rheumatic tendencies and nervous, hysterical temperament.

2. Unstable mental state constantly relapsing into profound **depression**; anxiety and fears of death, insanity, nature and extent of illness, etc.; loquacity; mental and physical restlessness; mental state alternating with physical.

3. **Utero-ovarian disorders**, with various reflex disturbances incidental thereto; e.g., severe headache occiput, vertex and/or behind the eyes, may extend to nape of neck and even spine; < motion > open air.

4. Rheumatic complaints esp. in the belly of muscles; often with persistent **muscular soreness**.

5. Pains sudden, sharp, lacinating; < touch motion; often assoc. with the voiding of profuse, pale urine with numbness.

6. Trembling and jerking of muscles < emotion, under pressure, e.g., when lying on the part; preventing sleep. Chorea.

7. Menses too painful, irregular and gen. scanty; pains < during the flow.

8. Ailments resulting from emotional causes esp. disappointments in the affections.

9. Left-sided complaints.

10. **Modalities**; < cold (except the headache) esp. cold damp weather; < during M.P.

Note : A valuable remedy to consult in disorders of pregnancy, and the puerperal state.

Keynote : Gloom.

CINCHONA OFFICINALIS

(China)

1. Stout, swarthy subjects; sallow, dingy-yellow complexion. Constitutions greatly **debilated by exhausting discharges esp. of body fluids.**

2. Patient apathetic, taciturn, despondent; dislikes company, > alone; irritability, fits of temper shallow (ctr. Nux–v,.); feels ill-used; over-sensitive to criticism.

3. **Hyperæsthesia** of the nervous system esp. **to touch.**

4. Alimentary disorders with **excessive flatulence** not > by eructations or dejections; voracious appetite yet even a light meal distresses owing to poor digestion; desires acids and fruits which <; < milk. Also complete anorexia.

5. Venous congestion followed by passive **hæmorrhages,** from any mucous orifice.

6. Anæmias with throbbing, bursting headaches, singing in the ears, weakness of sight, etc., and tendency to neuralgias esp. facial.

7. **Periodicity** of symptoms esp. of fevers and neuralgias; particularly if every other day.

8. Drawing or tearing pains in every limb and joint < rest > motion; body sore all over.

9. Discharges generally painless but exhausting.

10. Patient < cold and damp; autumn; **least touch** yet hard pressure >; < **least draught of air**; any mental or physical exertion; > warmth.

COCCULUS INDICUS

1. Fair women and children of weak, nervous temperament with tendency to spasmodic complaints; sensitive, romantic girls.

2. Patient cannot bear least contradiction; angry and offended at mere triffles; times passes too quickly.

3. Great lassitude of the whole body with trembling weakness.

4. Sensation of emptiness or **hollowness** in various organs.

5. Paralytic numbness esp. in hands and feet, various parts go to sleep.

6. Marked with or without nausea and vomiting complaints caused by or < **by motion of vehicles**, seasickness, etc.

7. Complaints (esp. hysteria) from **loss of sleep**, night watching, mental excitement, overwork, etc.

8. Abdominal distension with colic; no > from passing flatus; abdomen feels as if full of sharp sticks or stones.

9. M.P. premature and painful with extreme weakness; patient scarcely able to stand or talk.

10. Patient intolerant of all stimuli including touch and even fresh air; < mental and physical exertion even talking.

Keynote : **Paralytic Weakness**

COFFEA CRUDA

1. Tall, lean, stooping, dark-complexioned subjects sanguine, choleric temperament.

2. Generally cheerful disposition but subject to fits of temper though without spitefulness; variable moods.

3. **Hyperæsthesia of the special senses.**

4. Oversensitiveness to pain which seems insupportable driving to despair.

5. Ill-effects (esp. hysteria or insommnia) of sudden mental emotions, esp. pleasurable surprises.

6. **Sleeplessness** from excessive mental and physical excitement.

7. Headache, one-sided, as from nail driven into brain; increases throughout the day; < open air.

8. Nervous dyspepsia, sudden attack esp. about the M.P., > vomiting; agonizing yet patient otherwise well.

9. Toothache > only by ice-cold water.

10. **Modalities;** < cold and open air; excessive joy, etc.

Note : Coffee interferes with homoeopathic drug action.
Keynote : **Excitement.**

COLCHICUM AUTUMNALE

1. Rheumatic, gouty diathesis.

2. Patient ill-tempered and peevish; sufferings seems intolerable.

3. Oversensitiveness to all external impressions esp. odours.

4. Intense nausea, vomiting, even faintness from the **smell of cooking food** (Dig.); the sight or thought of food sickens.

5. Great **abdominal distension** from flatulence.

6. Autumnal complaints from damp, etc., esp. mucous colitis with discharge containing large quantities of small, white, shreddy particles; dysentery.

7. Sensation of burning or of icy coldness internally; with coldness of body surface even cold sweat.

8. **Arthritic complaints** esp. of small joints; powerlessness of the part; severe tearing pains, < motion, touch and at night; tendency to change locality esp. from left to right.

9. Dropsical conditions, particularly of cavities and internal organs. Kidney disorders with black, bloody albuminous urine.

10. **Modalities**; < damp, touch, motion, at night, mental exertion, and esp. from odours.

CONIUM MACULATUM

1. Old people esp. old maids and old bachelors, rigid muscular fibre; scrofulous or cancerous tendencies.

2. Lively, sanguine, disposition yet easily gets out of humour; moroseness; inability and disinclination for any mental effort, dreads being alone yet avoids society.

3. Chronic gland troubles; inflammations rather than growths; with **induration**; esp. of breasts; **after a blow**, etc.

4. **Vertigo on turning the head sideways** esp. to the left; on lying down or turning over in bed.

5. Spasmodic cough caused by dry spot in larynx, immediately on lying down (Hyos.); during pregnancy.

6. Eye diseases; intense photophobia out of all proportion to the objective signs of inflammation; < night > pressure, dark room.

7. Bladder troubles with great difficulty in voiding urine; the flow intermits.

8. Ill-effects of suppressed sexual desire, or of excessive indulgence; suppressed menses from putting hands in cold water.

9. **Sweating**, immediately **on falling asleep**, day or night, even **on closing the eyes** (ctr. Samb.).

10. Patient on the whole < cold; night; lying down, turning in bed; > in dark.

CUPRUM METALLICUM

1. Prostration with nervous trembling particularly as a result of mental strain and loss of sleep.

2. Patient ill-natured, angry, spiteful; mentally and physically oversensitive.

3. **Cramps, convulsions** and **spasmodic affections** generally. Clonic spasms beginning in fingers and toes. Epilepsies without any clear symptoms or where aura begins in knees and ascends.

4. Paralysis esp. of flexor muscles (extensors-Plb.); also of tongue.

5. Symptoms appear periodically and in groups.

6. Cholera and choleraic conditions; body, cold, skin blue, collapse: violent cramps abdomen and extremities.

7. **Repercussion of eruptions**; skin dusky, no rash but cerebral symptoms esp. convulsions.

8. Spasmodic respiratory troubles esp. whooping cough; long-continued paroxysms with difficult breathing, cyanosis and violent vomiting.

9. Gurgling sound as of water poured out a bottle when drinking or coughing.

10. **Modalities**;< cold air, contact, before M.P. nausea, vomiting and cough> drink of cold water (Caust.).

Note : Cuprum aceticum is to be preferred where a more rapid action is desired.
Keynote : **Spasms**.

FERRUM METALLICUM

1. Especially adapted to delicate, **anaemic women** with sanguine temperament; pseudo-plethora (cheeks flushed or easily flushed but mucous membranes pale).

2. Mental and physical **irritability**; intolerance of noise and pain; patient excitable, impulsive, changeable; solitude preferred.

3. Great debility with breathlessness; easily fatigued yet **must have gentle exercise.**

4. Local congestions with tendency to recurrent heamorrhages, esp. of upper air passages (Ferr–act., Ferr–p.).

5. Frequent attacks of hammering, pulsating h/a., often with hot head and cold extremities.

6. weak digestion; anorexia, sometimes alt. with bulimia; vomiting of food immediately after eating or coughing, or it lies in stomach all day and is then vomited just after midnight, aversion and < from eggs (rev. Calc.).

7. Irritability of rectum and bladder resulting in (a) diarrhoea of painless, watery or lienteric stools with flatulence **while eating and drinking**; (b) incontinence of urine particularly in women, spurts on coughing < day.

8. Menses premature, profuse, protracted; **flow pale, watery, debilitating.**

9. Muscular pains about the shoulder esp. left deltoid > gentle exertion; also cramps.

10. Patient chilly, < winter but extreme heat also <; > walking slowly about yet weakness obliges her to sit or lie down;> mental exertion; < after midnight; < sitting still.

GELSEMIUM SEMPERVIRENS

1. Neurotic, hysterical subjects esp. women and children. Nervous symptoms predominate in all complaints.

2. Mental and bodily lassitude; dull, drowsy, dizzy; wishes to be let alone; may be desire to throw herself from a height; or desire for expression in speech or writing with sense of increased power esp. of memory.

3. Complaints from mental emotions esp. **psychic diarrhoeas**.

4. Complete relaxation of the whole muscular system with entire motor paralysis; general tremor; **lack of muscular co-ordination.**

5. Spasmodic conditions or partial and local paralysis; in groups of muscles; professional neuroses (e.g., writer's cramp).

6. Dull, tired **headache** at base of brain: or beginning nape of neck or occiput and extending over head to one eye (gen. right) or both eyes; commences with blurred vision and acc. by vertige: < 10 a.m., > profuse urination.

7. **First stage of fevers**; asthenic tendency; patient languid and listless, wishes to be let alone; frequent, soft pulse; prostration, vertigo; more or less aching in back and limbs: little or no thirst; slight sweat; chills run up and down the back.

8. Acute catarrhal conditions with watery mucous discharges; much sneezing early a.m.. Influenzas with coryza.

40

9. Female disorders with severe neuralgic pains shooting into back, hips and down the thighs. Excellent at parturition in atonic conditions.

10. **Modalities**; < warm, moist, relaxing weather. Mental emotions; tobacco smoking; thinking of ailments; heat of sun and in summer yet locally heat often > pains; < motion except heart symptoms; > stimulants.

Keynote : **Paralysis.**

GRAPHITES

1. Scrofulous subjects esp. woman with tendency to unhealthy corpulence; sluggish, " pasty" habit. At climaxis.

2. Great sadness and despondency with inclination to weep esp. at hearing music: apprehension, mind dwells upon death. Children acute and impudent, laugh at reprimands.

3. Marked debility with anaemic conditions. Sexual debility from abuse.

4. Unhealthy skin; every injury suppurates.

   (a) Itching eruptions with oozing of corrosive, **transparent, honey-like fluid**; esp. about the ears, face or entire scalp; gen. < warmth.

   (b) Skin dry, nails become hard, thick, brittle; rhagades; excoriations; special affinity for scar tissue.

5. Glandular swellings and indurations.

6. Alimentary disorders > eating > warm milk, < cold drinks; dislikes sweets, animal food, fat, salt; tongue gen. clean.

7. Abdominal distension from flatulence with constipations; stools too large, lumpy covered with mucus or containing mucous shred; anus sore, even fissured.

8. Female complaints with delayed M.P.; flow gen. scanty but leucorrhoea of profuse, thin, white mucus, **in gushes day and night**; sometimes in place of menses.

9. Ear troubles: hears better in a noise (Nit–ac.), or on violent motion.

10. Patient chilly yet likes open air, < night, motion during and after M.P.

HEPAR SULPHUR

1. Scrofulous subjects, leucophlegmatic, inactive, slow; systems injured by mercury (first remedy).

2. Intense mental and physical **hypersensitiveness**; trifles make him angry; intolerance of pain, touch and even a draught of air.

3. General sourness and foetidness of all excretions, esp. in children.

4. Profuse and easy sweating esp. about the chest; day and night without relief.

5. Throbbing and sticking pains; sensation of splinter esp. in throat.

6. **Suppurative conditions** when pus is about to form or is formed; hastens suppuration (low potencies); staphylococcal infections (Silica-streptococcal); unhealthy skin, every injury suppurates; ulcers with foetid discharge, bleed easily, extremely **sensitive**.

7. Respiratory complaints, esp. from exposure to dry, cold air; **croupous conditions** with great hoarseness, whistling respirations, hard barking cough, or when cough becomes loose and rattling; cough < uncovering any part of body.

8. Atonic alimentary disorders; desire for vinegar and sour, pungent things and fat.

9. Atonic condition of rectum and bladder; (a) difficult defecation, caly-coloured stools; (b) difficult micturition,

slow, without force, urine drops vertically; bladder never thoroughly emptied.

10. Patient chilly,< **slightest draught**, > mild wet weather (Caust, Nux–V.); < night.

Note : Often indicated in slow, chronic conditions was well as acute states, esp. when complaints show no sign of clearing up.

IGNATIA AMARA

1. Nervous, hysterical women; dark hair and complexion; pale, wan, drawn appearance; disposition mild but easily excited; quick in perception, rapid in execution (ctr. Puls.)

2. **Rapid alternation of mental states** (Crocus., Puls.) with underlying condition of melancholy; **moodiness**; full of silent grief, **sits and sighs**; overdelicate conscience; sometimes angry but never ill-natured (see Cham., Nux–v); > alone but does not resent consolation.

3. Mental and physical **exhaustion from long-concentrated grief**, from worry or strain; from disappointed love, etc.

4. Hypersensitiveness, mental and physical; easily offended, intolerant of pain, etc.

5. Spasmodic affections originating in mental causes, < touch; chorea, convulsions, etc., in children, from fright, punishment or worms; globus hystericus.

6. Penetrating pains in small circumscribed spots, e.g. headache as of nail being driven in. > hard pressure, profuse urination, < movement.

7. Gastro-intestinal disorders; capricious appetite; sense of weakness and emptiness in stomach; dislikes stimulants; craves sour things; prefers cold food.

8. Constipation with excessive ineffectual urging felt more in upper abdomen; tendency to hæmorrhoids and prolapse; sharp stitches shoot up the rectum.

9. **Great contradictoriness of symptoms**, e.g. (a) grief excites laughter; (b) "sore" throat > swallowing esp. solids; (c) sinking in stomach not > eating; (d) piles > walking; (e) cough < coughing; (f) fevers with thirst only during chill; (g) headache > lying on the painful spot.

10. Patient chilly < out of doors, > heat except stomach symps.; < mental emotion, excitement; stimulants esp. coffee and **tobacco**; all strong sensory stimuli; pains gen. < movement.

Notes : Chronic-Nat–m. or Zinc.

Keynotes : **Contradictions, Coffee** and **tobacco** inimical to its action.

IODIUM

1. Scrofulous subjects; dark hair and eyes; dirty yellow skin; never fat; esp. children.

2. Patient excitable, restless, impulsive.

3. General sluggishness of patient and symptoms.

4. Great debility and **emaciation** in spite of voracious appetite; after shock or emotional strain; unaccountable sense of weakness and loss of breath on going upstairs.

5. Hypertrophy or atrophy of **glandular tissues**; usually painless; thyroid and mammæ specially affected.

6. Catarrhal affections of the mucous membranes esp. of the upper air passages. Membranous croup, early stage with feverishness, dry, hot skin, dry cough and dyspnæa (follows Acon.). Also T.B. infections.

7. Heart troubles with palpitation < least exertion, heart feels squeezed.

8. Chronic arthritis conditions after acute affections; intense pains at night; no swelling; after syphilis or mercury.

9. Salivation (Ip., Merc.).

10. Patient < warmth; wet weather; always > **out of doors; after or while eating.**

IPECACUANHA

1. The gastric symptoms predominate in nearly all complaints; **violent and persistent nausea not > vomiting.**

2. Morose irritability with pale, drawn face and hollow eyes encircled with dark rings. Children readily cry and scream and have vague, indefinite longings.

3. Alimentary disorders; aversion from all food with vomiting of tenacious, white glairy mucus; **tongue** usually **clean**; stomach feels as if "hanging relaxed"; after indulgence in rich, fat foods (Puls.) or sweets, ices, etc. (Ars.); salivation (Merc., Iod.).

4. Diarrhœas and dysentery; char. stools:

   (a) fermented, foamy like yeast, (b) grass green, mucous or watery, (c) slimy with more or less blood.

5. Respiratory complaints; violent dyspnœa with wheezing, anxious respiration, or dry, spasmodic cough; great accumulation of mucus (fine râles) yet nothing comes up.

6. Active or passive **hæmorrhages of bright arterial blood**; in gushes from all orifices.

7. Obstinate **Malarias** with no regularly defined stages; after abuse of quinine; will often bring out the true drug picture.

8. Pains as if bones all torn to pieces.

9. Intense irritation of the skin with uncontrollable desire to scratch.

10. Patient sensitive to every change of weather: <heat and cold, moist winds.

Keynote : **Nausea.**

KALIUM BICHROMICUM

1. Scrofulous, fat, fair subjects, disposed to catarrhal troubles.

2. No very characteristic mental symptoms.

3. **Catarrhal conditions** of any mucous membrane with **tough, tenacious, ropy discharges**, gen. yellow; also tough membranes on mucous surfaces.

4. **Ulcerations** esp. of mucous membranes; solitary, penetrating, **punched-out** appearance; usually with foetid, cheesy exudation: also extensive ulceration in the nose with **discharge of hard plugs** often leaving an eroded surface.

5. **Pains in small spots** (can be covered with point of finger): **wandering**, erratic, appear and disappear suddenly: periodic, neuralgic or rheumatic.

6. Alternating complaints: e.g. right-sided sick, headache and gastric symptoms; rheumatism and dysenteric trouble.

7. Tongue yellow-coated particularly at the base (Merc–i–f., Nat–s.): or (esp. in dysentery) smooth, red, glazed, dry and cracked.

8. Throat troubles with shooting pain extending into the ear; uvula oedematous with bladder-like appearance.

9. Croupous affections with hoarse, metallic cough. dyspnoea < lying down, char. expectoration causing gagging, etc., little or no fever; later stages.

10. Patient chilly, liable to take cold in the open air yet often < hot weather; < spring and early summer; morning esp. about 3 to 4 a.m.; skin symptoms> cold weather.

KALIUM CARBONICUM

1. Elderly persons with dark hair, **lax fibre**, inclined to obesity; feeble circulation; anaemic, broken-down constitutions; tendency to local congestions.

2. Mental slackness and weakness; disinclined to any exertion, peevish; unreasonable apprehensions; easily frightened; **intolerant of least touch** (esp. if unexpected) and of pain; dreads solitude.

3. Great debility with easy sweating and constant, **weary backache** > pressure.

4. Sharp, stitching pains, ‖ motion < lying affected side; char. region is between right hip and right knee on outer side of thigh.

5. Right-aided ailments.

6. **Bag-like swelling between eyebrows and lids**; a sagging of the tissues rather than oedema.

7. Catarrhal conditions of all mucous membranes; of respiratory tract with dryness and discharge of tenacious mucus, gen. scanty, difficult to dislodge; often with gagging and vomiting of ingesta.

8. Impaired digestion with great flatulent distension; abdomen sensitive to touch; constipation; capricious appetite with strong desire for sweet or sour things; assoc. neurasthenic conditions.

9. Chronic pelvic disorders in women; periods excessive; profuse leucorrhoea of mucus and pus; patient **feels sadly weak before M.P.**

10. Patient < cold, takes cold easily; open air, lying affected side; 2-4 a.m.; while eating and just after e.g. toothache;< coitus.

Note : Acute or chronic conditions.

KREOSOTUM

1. Tall, lean, dark-complexioned persons; poorly nourished and subject to bacterial infections; over-grown girls; children old-looking and wrinkled; women at post-climacteric period.

2. Children ill-humoured, peevish, cry for things which they push or throw away on receiving (Staph).

3. All secretions (esp. from mucous surfaces) **corrosive, acrid, very offensive, debilitating**. Septic discharges.

4. Violent **burning** pains, esp. in diseases with a gangrenous or **malignant tendency**.

5. Haemorrhagic diathesis; flow passive, dark, oozing.

6. Painful dentition: teeth begin to decay as soon as they appear; scorbutic of the mouth: pyorrhoea.

7. Persistent vomiting: of sweetish water; of undigested food in large quantities long after meals: often sympathetic (pregnancy, etc.).

8. Female disorders: periods premature, profuse, protracted; **flow only on lying down**; intermitting; between periods-leucorrhoea, offensive, acrid causing itching and burning to the parts < scratching; stains linen yellow; with debility.

9. Urinary troubles; sudden urging; copious, pale discharge; can only micturate when lying down; incontinence in children during first sleep (Sep.) which is very profound.

10. **Modalities**; < cold weather, cold air, cold bathing; < rest esp. when lying.

Note : Inimical to Carb–v.

F - 5

LAC CANINUM

1. Nervous, restless, highly sensitive temperament.

2. Patient **forgetful**, absent-minded; drops letters and words in writing; cannot concentrate; intense despondency-a **chronic "blue" condition**; attacks of rage; fears solitude, death, insanity, falling down stairs, etc.

3. **Symptoms erratic; change from side to side** every few hours or days; apt to begin and end with M.P.

4. Throat complaints; sensitive to touch externally (Lach.): pains extend to the ears; < empty swallowing.

5. **Shining, glazed appearance of lesions**; e.g. diphtheritic deposit, ulcers, etc.

6. Sinking feeling at epigastrium; usually not > eating.

7. Female disorders. Periods premature. Profuse, flow bright, viscid, stringy, in gushes. Breasts painful, inflamed, < towards evening and from least jar; must hold them firmly when going up or down stairs. Useful when necessary to dry up the milk.

8. Hyperaesthesia of the sexual organs.

9. Intense backache across supra-sacral region extending to right natis and down right sciatic nerve; spine very sensitive to touch and pressure.

10. **Modalities**: < at M.P.; often < lying left side.

Note : Acts best in single dose.

LACHESIS MUTUS

1. Dark, phlegmatic subjects; or women with red hair and freckled complexion,.esp. at **climaxis**; also broken-down constitutions.

2. Extreme alternations, mind and sensorium, (a) Mental activity with almost prophetic perception; ecstasy; **loquacity** with rapid change of subject esp. when delirious; hurry and flurry; delusion of voices, etc. (b) Depression with anxiety; patient silent, suspicious; jealous; weak memory, writing mistakes; deranged time sense; self-consciousness and selfishness.

3. Hyperaesthesia of the senses; of body surface; nervous **intolerance of** touch, pressure and **constriction**, even of clothing, esp. about throat and abdomen.

4. Marked aggravation of all complaints from sleep; patient **sleeps into an attack**; sleep disturbed by frightful dreams, of dead and dying people, of suffocation, etc.

5. All distressing symptoms are > onset of discharges; e.g. at **M.P. always** > **during flow**.

6. Ailments **left-sided or travel from left to right**; yet a special affinity for the appendix.

7. Adynamic fevers with low, muttering delirium; face purplish, besotted-looking, dropped jaw; offensive breath; tremors esp. of the tongue which is protruded with difficulty; **haemorrhages** of dark, decomposed blood.

8. Septic states; malignant ulcerations and suppuration; with offensive discharges and **bluish**, livid appearance; gangrene.

9. Tremors, cramps, spasms and even convulsions.

10. **Modalities**; < heat esp. heat of sun; **muggy weather**; must have air; < spring; **throat symptoms** < **hot drinks** and empty swallowing or liquids < than solids.

Note : The great trio of remedies for women at climaxis–Lach., Sep. and Sulph.

LEDUMPALUSTRE

1. Rheumatic, gouty diathesis; old people; constitutions suffering from abuse of alcohol.

2. Discontent and peevishness.

3. Alternating complaints, e.g. haemoptysis and rheumatism; symptoms appearing diagonally esp. upper left and lower right (Ant–t., Agar., Stram.; upper right lower left-Brom., Medorr., Phos., etc.).

4. Contusions esp. about the eye; patient bruises easily; long-remaining discoloration after injuries. **Punctured wounds** including insect bites esp. of mosquitoes (locally and internally).

5. **Rheumatic and arthritic complaints**; beginning lower limbs and ascending; first feet then hands; small joints mostly affected; painful nodosities; rarely useful if heat and swelling; pains < motion, night, **warmth of bed**; sometimes > only when holding feet in ice-water.

6. Skin eruptions; papular, eczematous; in habitual drunkards; esp. face, forehead; chronic eruptions with violent itching esp. feet and ankles < scratching, warmth of bed.

7. Emphysemas and bronchitis of the aged < hot rooms; spasmodic coughs.

8. Haemorrhages esp. of bright-red blood; intraocular heamorrhage.

9. Pains sticking, tearing or throbbing; rapidly change locality.

10. Patient lacks vital heat; **always cold** yet pains < heat esp. of bed, > cool applications.

LILIUM TIGRINUM

1. Women with utero-ovarian disorders and ailments incidental thereto.

2. Profound melancholic state esp. religious, < consolation fears solitude, insanity, incurability, or some impending disease of calamity; crazy feeling on vertex.

3. Patient listless yet restless; **must keep busy**; aimless, hurried motion, often to suppress sexual desire.

4. Persistent **bearing down** in abdomen and pelvis as though all the organs would escape; wants to support vulva with the hands. Uterine displacements (all forms, esp. versions); pressure against rectum and bladder results in constipation or constant desire to defecate and urinate. Shooting pains (ctr. Sep.).

5. Menstrual disorders; **flow only on moving about.**

6. Pulsations over whole body. Pains in small spots; constantly shifting.

7. Inability to walk on uneven ground.

8. Reflex heart symptoms; pain, fluttering, palpitation, with sensation as if heart alternately grasped and relaxed (Cact.).

9. Ailments principally left-sided.

10. **Modalities** gen. < hot weather, > fresh air; < evening and night;> keeping busy.

LYCOPODIUM CLAVATUM

1. Patient **intellectually keen but physically weak**; emaciation upper part of body; sedentary habit; mentally absorbed; complexion often sallow; prematurely old in appearance. Children precocious, weakly.

2. Mental powers failing; fatigue and forgetfulness uses wrong words, etc.; hypochondriasis with irritability; emotionally sensitive; lachrymose; apprehensive of the future; **lacks self-confidence** yet "gets through"; dislikes company yet dreads solitude; thwomen dread of man.

3. **Chronic gastro-intestinal disorders**; general sourness of alimentary tract; appetite good but a few mouthfuls satiate; **flatulence** excessive, much borborygmus, > dejections; craves sweets, delicacies; dislikes oysters and often meat; < coffee, wine, smoking, onions; constipation predominates.

4. Uric acid diathesis; **red sand in urine**, child cries before micturition; or increased quantity of pale urine.

5. Dryness of skin (esp. palms) and mucous membranes; stoppage of nose with discharge of crusts or elastic plugs.

6. Fan-like motion of the alae nasi, of a twitching nature and independent of respiration (in respiratory troubles- Ant–t.).

7. One foot hot (usually the right) the other cold.

8. Irritability after uninterrupted nap.

9. Complaints **right-sided** or travel form right to left.

10. **Modalities**;< both extremes of temperature but esp. heat; heat of exertion; < **4-8 p.m.**, sometimes continuing later (Hell.); sleep; constriction; > in open air esp. with uncovering and gentle motion; gastro-intestinal symptom > warmth.

Note : In deep-seated, progressive, chronic diseases.

MAGNESIUM CARBONICUM

1. Subjects of lax fibre esp. children; nervous temperament constitutions worn out by long strain and anxiety.

2. Irritable disposition.

3. Mental and physical sensitiveness.

4. Sour smell of whole body; all excretions tend to sourness.

5. Neuralgias with lightning-like pains; of face < left side, < at night; insupportable during rest; esp. during pregnancy.

6. Alimentary complaints; acid dyspepsia, even vomiting; of pregnancy; inordinate craving for meat in children; < milk, cabbage, potatoes and other gross foods.

7. Diarrhoea preceded by colic; **stools green, frothy, like scum of frog pond**; milk passes undigested; white floating lumps like tallow.

8. Menstrual disorders; **flow only or < at night or when lying down** (Am–m., Kreos., rev. Lil–t.); ailments of pregnancy.

9. Epileptiform spasms.

10. Modalities; < change of temperature; at M.P.; warmth of bed but> warn air; < every three weeks; abdominal pains > bending over.

MEDORRHINUM

1. Deep-seated sycotic chronic affections esp. after maltreated or suppressed gonorrhoea, when best selected remedy fails to relieve or permanently improve.

2. Patient **lachrymose**; cannot speak without weeping; always anticipating events, even death; memory weak; mentally sensitive; irritable, impatient.

3. Intensely **restless and fidgety legs and feet** (Zinc.): subjective trembling all over.

4. **Burning of hands and feet**; wants them uncovered and fanned (Lach., Sulph).

5. Rheumatic and arthritic complaints of sycotic origin; puffy swelling and painful stiffness of joints, **esp. knuckles;** constricting pains; soreness all over.

6. **Insatiate cravings**; for liquor, salt, sweets, fruits, etc.; usually constipation.

7. **Nocturnal enuresis**; passes enormous quantities of ammoniacal, high-coloured urine in bed every night.

8. Female pelvic disorders esp. if symptoms tend to malignancy with or without sycotic origin; menorrhagia and metrorrhagia, flow profuse, dark,, clotted.

9. Collapsed state; wants to be fanned; skin and sweat cold yet throws off covering; craves fresh air.

10. **Modalities**; < **daylight to sunset** (rev. Syph.); < heat, covering, thunder-storm, motion; > **at seashore** (rev. Nat–m.);> lying on the stomach esp. in respiratory complaints.

MERCURIUS (VIVUS, OR SOLUBILIS)

1. Light-haired subjects of lax fibre; earthy or dirty-yellow, rough complexion. Anti-syphilitic, second stage.

2. Mental slowness but states changeable; (a) memory and will power deficient; answers questions slowly; despondency; (b) hurry and anxiety; loquacity, esp. in delirium; time passes slowly.

3. Weakness and weariness in all the limbs with pronounced tremor, esp. of hands; goes on to paresis and paralysis; with great restlessness.

4. **Suppurative conditions**; low potencies hasten, high potencies abort suppuration; of gland; also eruptions of many kinds.

5. Superficial ulcerations; spreading, everted edges, cheesy base, readily bleed, discharge excoriating; esp. about the mouth and throat.

6. Ptyalism: profuse, soapy, stringy saliva; foetid metallic taste. **Tongue swollen, flabby, showing teeth imprints**, coated gen. moist yet interse thirst present.

7. All mucous membranes have free secretion of slimy muco-pus, often with ulceration; discharge first thin, excoriating then thicker and more bland; gen. greenish; naso-pharyngeal region and colon esp. affected; dysenteric **stools with much blood** and tenesmus, not > stool.

8. Profuse sweating without > esp. in fevers.

9. Bone diseases with boring pains < night; exostosis.

10. Patient < both heat and cold; at **every change** esp. to damp weather; **all night, warmth of bed**; lying right side; joints also < **touch**, pressure and movement.

Notes : In skin affections Merccurius Solubis is to be preferred. Merccurius Cyanatus invaluable in diphtheria. Merccurius bi–iodatus in left sided-Merccurius Protoiodatus, in right-sided throat conditions. Incompatible with Silica.

MEZEREUM

1. Light-haired, irresolute persons of phlegmatic temperament; often scrofulous or syphilitic.

2. Hypochondriasis; indifferent to everything and every one; angry at trifles but soon sorry.

3. Vesicular and **pustular eruptions**, esp. after vaccination; copious exudation of thick pus over which **tough scabs form**; appear esp. about the face and head; child scratches till covered with blood; intolerable itching and burning < scratching, at night and form heat.

4. Ulcerations with much thick scabbing under which pus collects; ulcers sensitive, bleed easily and are often surrounded with burning, itching vesicles.

5. Periosteal pains and infflammations; of long bones esp. tibiae; burning or flying, stitching pains, < damp, at night in bed; caries; exostoses, tumours soften from within.

6. **Neuralgias** esp. following eruptions (e.g. zona) or mercurialism; particularly of face involving eye, cheek and teeth; severe, tearing pains with local soreness; followed by numbness.

7. Toothache with caries; teeth feel blunt and elongated.

8. Gastric disorders with burning pains and pressure (Ars.) even ulceration; patient craves fat; constipation usual.

9. Ailments usually one-sided.

10. **Modalities**; < **night, warmth of bed**, touch; cold air and cold washing.

NATRIUM CARBONICUM

1. Anaemic, emaciated subjects with pale face, blue-ringed eyes, dilated pupils, etc.

2. Intense melancholy and apprehension; mental slackness and **inability to think**; irritability; dislikes society esp. men; easily startled.

3. Great debility; heaviness of whole body; short walk greatly fatigues.

4. Ailments from **exposure to sun**, also artificial light; chronic effects of sunstroke or overstudy.

5. Gastric disorders with great acidity; large appetite; < after vegetable diet, starchy foods; discomfort > while eating.

6. Bearing down pains in female pelvic organs.

7. Chronic catarrhal conditions of all mucous membranes; gen. with copious secretion of thick mucus, usually yellowish-green; much nasal mucus passes through the mouth; < daytime, slightest draught, > sweating.

8. Ankles weak, give way when walking; easy dislocation and springing.

9. Skin dry, rough, chapped esp. dorsi of hands and feet; chronic dry eczemas.

10. Patient < during thunderstorm (from electrical changes not timidity); **excessive summer heat** yet dislikes open air; < **mental exertion**, music; between meals.

NATRIUM MURIATICUM

1. Cachectic, anaemic subjects; pale, earthy or yellowish, greasy-looking complexion; children emaciated (esp. about the neck) and old in appearance; debility from loss of vital fluids.

2. Great depression; lachrymose yet irritable esp. at small, non-essential noises; seems to desire but is markedly < **consolation**; dislikes company, > alone; emotionally sensitive to music; memory weak with inability to concentrate; hysteria, affections beyond control.

3. **Headaches**, chronic, hammering, periodic, blinding; **from sunrise to sunset**, < motion > semi-recumbent position, face pale or only slightly diffused; esp. in anaemic girls and women.

4. Condition of mucous membranes:- (a) chronic; dryness with ulcerations or cracks; e.g. of alimentary canal with constipation, dry, crumbling stools, and sore, fissured anus; (b) acute; **free watery discharges**, often coarse, frothy mucus esp. from upper respiratory tract.

5. Good appetite yet emaciation; inordinate **craving for salt** (Phos.) dislike to fats and bread; > going without regular meals.

6. **"Mapped" tongue** (patchy appearance) with sense of dryness and violent thirst.

7. Skin; (a) chronic; dryness with fissures, corns, warts, hangnails, etc., (b) acute; eczematous eruptions, raw

surface, acrid, watery discharge, esp. at scalp margin; acne; urticaria, after violent exercise; **hydroa** on lips or tongue, esp. during colds or intermittents.

8. Backache; severe, sacro-lumbar;> pressure, e.g. lying on something hard; often assoc. with delayed M.P. and bearing-down pains.

9. Inability to micturate in the presence of others.

10. **Modalities**; < heat esp. close room, must have air though apt to feel chilly and take cold; < 9-11 a.m.; salt; at seaside, etc.; mental exertion;> loose clothing.

Notes : Chronic of Ignatia amara and Bryonia alba. Should not be given during a fever paroxysm.

NATRIUM SULPHURICUM

1. Hydrogenoid constitutions; subjects with sycotic history.

2. Depression; **lively music saddens**; satiety of life; irritability, esp. when spoken to; inability to think.

3. Mental traumatism; mental effects of blow on the head, etc.

4. Catarrhas of mucous membranes with free discharge of **greenish-yellow muco-pus**; sometimes bloody.

5. Diarrhoeas, esp. chronic; **on first rising and moving about** in a.m.; sudden urging, gushing, with much flatus; fluid, yellow stools; < after vegetables and farinaceous foods.

6. Loose coughs with soreness and pain through left chest esp. lower lobe left lung; > sitting up and holding chest with both hands.

7. Spinal meningitis with violent crushing, gnawing pain at base of brain; delirium; opisthotonos.

8. Rheumatic complaints in sycotic or hydrogenoid patients always < damp; restless, must change position but little or no >.

9. Warty growths on skin and mucous membranes; granules on eyelids like small blisters.

10. **Modalities;< all forms of damp**; sea air; by day; lying left side; > open air.

NITRICUM ACIDUM

1. Dark-complexioned, thin subjects of rigid fibre who readily catch cold; naturally or prematurely old people with general weakness and emaciation; sycotic or mercurio-syphilitic states, or advanced cases of phthisis.

2. Depression and irritability with vindictiveness; patient excitable; anxious about his disease or past troubles.

3. Ulcerations, fissures, condylomata, warts, etc., esp. at all **muco-cutaneous orifices**, with easy though usually slight bleeding.

4. Cutting **or pricking pains** and sensations **as from splinters**, esp. on touching the part.

5. Thin, offensive excoriating discharges; sometimes purulent, dirty yellowish green.

6. Ptyalism; offensive odour of breath, etc., with diseased conditions of the mouth in general.

7. Haemorrhages of bright red blood, generally scanty.

8. Urine **scanty, dark brown and strong-smelling** (Benz–ac.) ; often cold when passed.

9. Ailments predominantly right-sided.

10. **Modalities**; < cold; change of weather; night; touch, etc. > while riding in vehicles.

NUX MOSCHATA

1. Woman and children of nervous, hysterical temperament; old people.

2. Rapid change of moods; absent-mindedness, loss of memory; thoughts vanish while writing; talking, etc.; sense of double personality; visionary dreamy states; indifference.

3. Hypersensitiveness to all external stimuli.

4. Great **drowsiness** with nearly all complaints; dizziness and **disposition to faint**.

5. Marked **dryness** of all mucous membranes esp. of mouth, tongue and throat without thirst; also dry skin which rarely sweats.

6. Enormous **distension** of abdomen during or just after every meal; without much pain; everything seems to turn to gas.

7. Complaints of pregnancy; e.g. hysteria, toothache, vomiting, cough, diarrhoea.

8. Spasmodic affections; tonic followed by clonic spasms.

9. Haemorrhages, esp. menorrhagia of thick, dark blood.

10. Patient < cold, wet and windy weather; cold food, water and washing; least emotional excitement; > warmth generally.

NUX VOMICA

1. Dark, sallow, spare subjects of passionate temperament; sedentary brain workers; chronic dyspeptics addicted to stimulants; victims of drug habits, drastic medicines, excesses, etc.

2. Hypochondriasis with **irascibility** and impatience; spiteful and malicious or sullen and surly, thinks everyone is against him; melancholy > alone esp. from relatives; "spasmodic" homicidal or suicidal impulses; precise, ardent but overbearing; dread of, and incapacity for literary work.

3. Mental and physical **hypersensitiveness** (even fainting) to external stimuli; also to pain, trifling ailments, etc.

4. **Gastric disorders** from atony; hunger yet no desire for food; distension and **discomfort an hour or so after meals** with nausea; taste, eructations, vomit, etc., **all sour** or bitter, "if only could vomit would be better", assoc. "bilious" morning headaches; craving for condiments and sour or bitter things; likes fat.

5. Habitual constipation; **frequent but ineffectual desire for stools**, or small quantities passed at each attempt (from spasmodic peristalsis); blind or bleeding piles; stool temporarily >.

6. M.P. premature, profuse, protracted with bearing-down pains, nausea in a.m., chilliness and attacks of faintness.

7. Drowsiness during evening, **wakeful at 3-4. a.m.**, but later falls into heavy, unrefreshing sleep; awakes late tired and worn out. Always > undisturbed sleep.

8. Convulsions with consciousness; tetanic rigidity < external stimuli esp. touch; also violent local muscular contractions.

9. In fevers patient must be **covered in every stage**-chill, heat and sweat; cannot move or uncover without being chilly.

10. Patient **very chilly**, < winter, open air and draughts; dry weather; mental exertion; anger; mornings; after eating;> warmth; mild, damp weather.

Notes : Nux vomica acts during repose of mind and body; dose a few hours before retiring. Sep. often its chronic. Zinc. is inimical.

Keynote : **Irritable tension.**

OPIUM

1. Children and old people of lax fibre; fair-complexioned; also indicated in drunkards.

2. Ailments from fright esp. where fear still remains; fear of impending death.

3. All complaints with great sopor; **no pain, no complaint, no desires.**

4. Low types of fever; mild delirium, constant talking, eyes wide open, face red and puffed; thinks he is not at home; later-unconscious, eyes glassy, half closed, pupils contracted, face pale.

5. Cerebal congestions (esp. in drunkards); heavy, stupid sleep; bloated, red face; eyes blood-shot and half closed; **stertorous breathing**; skin covered with hot sweat.

6. Partial or complete local paralysis; paralysis of brain from sudden retrocession of acute exanthema.

7. **Inactivity of all organs** esp. alimentary tract; e.g. constipation, no desire for stool; impacted faeces, incarcerated flatus; stools hard, round, black; after long use of purgatives and enemas; also involuntary black, offensive stools. Retention of urine with full bladder.

8. No vital reaction; **want of susceptibility to well chosen remedies.**

9. Insomnia, bed feels so hot patient cannot lie upon it.

10. **Modalities**; < heat; during and after sleep; stimulants; while sweating.

Keynote : **Inertia.**

PETROLEUM

1. Fair-complexioned subjects who take cold easily.

2. Irritability and quarrelsomeness; trifles offend.

3. Low fevers with delirium; patient imagines there is **another person in the bed**; that he is double; that two babies are in the bed beside her.

4. Occipital vertigo or headache with pressure and heaviness like lead.

5. Ailments from riding in vehicles, etc; seasickness.

6. Gastric complaints > **by constant eating**; nausea in the morning with accumulation of water in the mouth.

7. Diarrhoea (lienteric) and dysentery **only in the day-time**; gushing; from taking cold or eating cabbage; from suppressed skin eruptions; discharges offensive.

8. Skin complaints; (a) **skin dry, rough and cracked**; sore and bleeding; < winter, washing, contact of clothes, etc.; **esp. tips of fingers**; painful, itching chilblains; (b) herpetic and eczematous eruptions; parts fiery-red and raw, oozing a thick gelatinous fluid; violent itching and burning; may go on to formation of thick crusts oozing pus.

9. Chronic rheumatism with great stiffness of joints; cracking sounds on movement.

10. **Modalities**;< before and during thunder-storm; **in winter**.

PHOSPHORICUM ACIDUM

1. Debilitated constitutions; pale sickly complexion, eyes sunken and surrounded by blue rings. Young people who grow too fast.

2. **Listlessness and apathy**; patient disinclined to talk; stupefied by grief.

3. Great debility from long- continued, depressing emotional causes, after violent acute diseases or **loss of vital fluids**; neurasthenias of sexual origin.

4. Adynamic fevers with complete apathy and stupor yet patient fully conscious if aroused; abdomen tympanitic; tongue has red streak down center widening in front; involuntary stools; haemorrhages of dark blood.

5. Headaches with crushing pain on vertex; < least noise esp. music;< motion> lying down; also headaches from eye-strain.

6. Chronic diarrhoeas, **painless, not-debilitating**; pale or whitish stools.

7. Polyuria esp. at night; urine clear and watery or like milk (excess of phosphates).

8. Interstitial inflammations of bones; pains as if scraped with a knife.

9. Weakness in the chest esp. from talking or coughing (Stann.).

10. Patient gen. > sleep; pains usually > motion.

PHOSPHORUS

1. Tall, slender subjects; fair or red hair; sometimes complexion pale, lemon-yellow tint; quick, lively sensitive temperament. Young people who grow too rapidly; narrow-chested, inclined to stoop; esp. if anaemic or T.B. tendency; blue rings and much puffiness around the eyes.

2. Indifference (even towards family); talks little or only in monosyllables; occasional fits of excitement and enthusiasm; disinclined to mental and physical exertion; slow; depressed, weary of life, **full of fears** esp. < alone, dark and thunder; gloomy forebodings; craves sympathy.

3. **Neurasthenic condition**; weakness and weariness with tremblings, often from loss of vital fluids; general restlessness and fidgetiness; hypersensitiveness to all external stimuli and to psychical influences.

4. **Burning** sensations **in spots**, esp. dorsal region of spine; intense heat running up the back into head (rev. Pic–ac.).

5. Haemorrhages, bright-red blood; haemophilia; patient bruises easily; purpura with abdominal symptoms.

6. **Emptiness** (weakness) in various localities; esp. **of entire abdomen about 11a.m.** which < all other symptoms; far, sudden noises, etc. "strike patient in the stomach".

7. Gastric symptoms; hunger, must eat often esp. during night; **craves salt**, cold food and drink; great thirst but water vomited soon as warm in the stomach; unchanged food

regurgitated in mouthfuls; nausea from putting hands in hot water.

8. Diarrhoeas; **very forcible**; as soon as anything enters rectum; gen. painless but debilitating; stool contains white, sago-like particles; **anus feels open**; involuntary oozing. Constipation; long slender, hard stools.

9. Wide use in acute and chronic diseases of **respiratory tract**; much tightness or rawness; **oppression** as of heavy weight on the chest; coughs < going from warm into cold air, using the voice, eating, drinking, etc.; lying left side. Right-sided lobar pneumonias.

10. **Modalities**;< cold (except stomach and head symptoms);< every change of weather; **during thunder**; twilight to midnight;> lying down but < **lying left side**;> sleep.

Notes : Incompatible with Causticum. Long and deep acting remedy but often "hangs fife" at first. Checks post-anaesthetic vomiting; best given twelve hours before.

PHYTOLACCA DECANDRA

1. Rheumatic subjects esp. if mercurio-syphilitic history.

2. Indifference to life; feels sure will die.

3. Aching, bruised soreness in all the muscles esp. of head, back and limbs; patient must move yet motion <.

4. Pains, "rheumatic", shooting, lancinating; flying like electric shocks; rapidly shift locality; < motion, damp, at night.

5. **Throat** complaints; parts dark red; intense **burning and dryness**; cannot drink hot fluids; great pain at root of tongue when swallowing; pains shooting through both ears.

6. **Mammary disorders**; inflammation, breasts full, **hard, stony, painful**; may go on to suppuration with abscesses, fistulae or gaping, angry ulcers; discharge of watery or foetid pus. Pains radiate from nipples all over body esp. when child nurses; nipples sensitive. Sore and fissured. Lumps in the breast (high potencies).

7. Difficult dentition and accompanying ailments; irresistible desire to bite the teeth or gums together.

8. Inflammation and swelling of bones and glands in general.

9. Right-sided pains and complaints.

10. **Modalities**; < damp weather; always < night most symptoms > lying down; open air.

Notes : Occupies a position between Bryonia alba and Rhus–tox.; will often cure when either fail though apparently well indicated.

PLATINA

1. Sanguine, thin, dark-haired women of rigid fibre.

2. Alternating mental states; peculiar **arrogance** and **illusionary greatness**; sometimes impulses to injure or even kill persons previously cared for (often distresses patient). Melancholy mood; life wearisome yet fears death which she thinks near; long sulks; vexation at trifles.

3. Physical and mental symptoms alternate.

4. Pains constricting, cramp-like; gradually increase to a severe point then gradually decrease (rev. Bell.).

5. Painful numbness of various parts often assoc. with the pains.

6. Chronic pelvic conditions in women; with bearing-down pains; M.P. premature, profuse; **flow dark, clotted**; great **hypersensitiveness of genitalia**; cannot bear touch even of clothing: violent sexual desire.

7. Reflex symptoms, esp. mental and nervous, from utero-ovarian disorders.

8. Obstinate constipation from inertia; **stools adhesive** like soft clay; abdomen retracted: flatulent colic; sense of weakness in abdomen.

9. Right-sided ailments (left-sided–Dr. Wheeler).

10. **Modalities**;< heat; evening and night; sitting or standing; fasting; > motion in the open air.

PLUMBUM METALLICUM

1. Persons with sallow, greasy-looking complexion, dark, "bilious" individuals with **sunken cheeks; cadaverous appearance.**

2. Intellectual torpor; apathy; loss of memory; unable to find proper word; hypochondriasis with irritability; religious melancholia; thinks much about physical health esp. his digestion.

3. Anaemia with great lassitude; **excessive and rapid emaciation of parts.**

4. Spasms esp. of sphincters; cramps, convulsions; tremors; going on to general or partial paralysis with hypereasthesia esp. if preceded by characteristic pains or mental derangement. Wrist-drop.

5. Arthralgic and neuralgic pains in trunk and limbs.

6. **Distinct blue line along gum margins**; foetid breath. Yellow tongue, sweetish taste.

7. **Excruciating colic**, sensation as if abdomen retracted to the spine, "as if drawn in by a string" pain radiates to all parts of the body.

8. Constipation; **stools painful, hard, lumpy, dark**, "like sheep's dung"; with spasms of sphincter ani.

9. Marked dryness of the skin; entire lack of perspiration.

10. **Modalities**;< night, motion;> hard pressure.

Note : A slow but deep-acting remedy.

PODOPHYLLUM PELTATUM

1. Sallow-complexioned subjects; lax fibre; "bilious" temperament Children.

2. Depression about his disease, etc.; thinks he will die.

3. Alternating complaints; e.g. winter headache alt. summer diarrhoea.

4. Difficult dentition; moaning and grinding of teeth at night; intense desire to press gums together (Phyt.); **head hot and rolling from side to side** (Bell., Hell.); often with diarrhoea as 6.

5. Hepatic troubles; torpidity of liver with white or yellow-coated tongue, jaundice, etc.; constant **desire to rub or shake liver region** with the hands.

6. Acute or chronic **diarrhœas; painless** or with colic; various stools but gen. profuse, watery, foetid and exhausting; with tendency to hæmorrhoids or prolapse of rectum; < early morning, continues during forenoon, followed later in the day by a natural stool (Aloe); < eating or drinking; dentition diarrhoea of dirty water soaking through napkin; while being washed.

7. Prolapse of rectum or of uterus esp. from over-straining or lifting, with aching and bearing down pains.

8. Intermittent or remittent fevers where bilious symptoms predominate; violent chills then intense fever with great **loquacity**, followed by sleep; attacks come on at 7 a.m.

9. Right-sided complaints, e.g. ovarian pains.

10. **Modalities**; < hot weather; early morning.

PSORINUM

1. Psoric subjects; coarse, dry or greasy skin, nervous, restless temperament; pale, delicate, sickly children.

2. Great mental depression; anxiety with evil forebodings; fears will die; religious melancholy; frightful dreams; children good all day, cry all night.

3. In chronic cases when **well selected remedies fail to relieve** or permanently improve (in acute-Sulph.); great debility remaining after acute diseases.

4. **Body and all excretions have a horrible odour.**

5. Feels unusually well the day before an attack.

6. Dry, scaly eruptions disappear in summer return in winter; itching < warmth of bed and when body gets warm; repeated outbreaks; ailments from suppressed skin diseases; skin dry, inactive, rarely sweats except after acute diseases when sweat profuse > all sufferings.

7. Marked tendency to quinsy, hay fever and to sprains.

8. **Always hungry**; esp. middle of night, must eat; during headache > while eating.

9. Asthmas, etc. > lying down and keeping arms stretched far apart.

10. Patient **very sensitive to cold air**, change of weather, esp. < stormy weather; restless for days before **thunder-storm.**

PULSATILLA NIGRICANS

1. Persons with sandy hair, pale face, blue eyes, sedentary habit; slow, gentle, yielding, emotional temperament. Anæmic, chlorotic women; girls in their teens; often overdosed with iron, quinine and other "tonics"; subject to styes and varicosis.

2. **Great changeableness** both of patient and symptoms; prevailing mood of melancholy with tearfulness, weeps when detailing symptoms; self-pity; likes consolation sentimental esp. at twilight; full of strange ideas esp. in the religious sphere; submissive yet at times peculiarly obstinate, easily upset, etc., never pugnacious (ctr. Nux–v.).

3. Acute or sub-acute catarrhal conditions; discharges copious, creamy, **yellow or greenish-yellow, thick and bland** (leucorrhœa may be acrid).

4. Drawing, tearing pains; erratic, **rapidly shift locality**; with characteristic modalitites; acc. by chilliness yet cool air >.

5. **Thirstlessness** with nearly all complaints yet dryness of the mouth esp. a.m. (rev. Merc.).

6. Gastro-intestinal complaints from overloading the stomach; from eating **rich foods, fat, pork,** etc.; from fruit, cold things, ices; thickly coated white tongue; hates fat, likes sour things and things not good for her; diarrhoetic stools, very changeable- **no two stools alike.**

84

7. Various **menstrual disorders**; periods irregular, gen. delayed and scanty; flow intermits and only or < during daytime; derangements at puberty in chlorotic girls; amenorrhoea esp. from getting feet wet, also ailments resulting therefrom. A valuable remedy during pregnancy and after.

8. One-sided complaints esp. sweats.

9. Sleeplessness; evening and first part of night but sleeps late into the morning; weaker the longer she lies (ctr. Nux–v.).

10. **Modalities**; < warmth esp. **warm rooms**; > **gentle motion in cool open air**, yet may complain of chilliness; > cold applications; < **twilight** to mid-night; lying left or **painless side**, abuse of tea.

Notes : Silica the chronic remedy in nearly all complaints.

Keynote : **Instability.**

RHUS TOXICODENDRON

1. Adapted to the rheumatic diathesis.

2. Great sadness and apprehension with inclination to weep; < at night, in the house > out of doors.

3. Sub-acute and chronic rheumatism and rheumatoid affections with the characteristic modalitites; pains as if the bones were scraped with a knife; also paralytic weakness with numbness and heaviness esp. lower limbs.

4. **Pains < rest, < on beginning to move, > continued motion**, temp. > change of position; pains return if movement continues to point of fatigue.

5. Muscle or tendon **strains**, stiffness or soreness esp. from overlifting or overreaching; < or grasping.

6. Adynamic fevers with mild delirium and stupefaction yet regular and persistent **restlessness** (from physical causes); red, dry, cracked, coated tongue, **triangular red tip**; sordes; stools loose, yellowish-brown, offensive, or bloody, frothy, sometimes involuntary during sleep, with great exhaustion.

7. All secretions and excretions acrid and foetid.

8. Complaints chiefly right-sided.

9. Acute skin diseases; **eczematous eruptions**, surface raw, excoriated; thick crusts oozing and offensive; much burning and itching; rubbing increases the eruption. Erysipelas, vesicular, phlegmonous; parts dark red; esp. of scalp, face and genitals.

10. **Modalities**; < cold esp. **cold, wet weather**, cold winds; getting wet esp. after overheating; before storms; after midnight; **during and after rest**.

Note : Apis inimical.

SANGUINARIA CANADENSIS

1. Young people; women at climaxis.

2. No marked mentals except hopeful state in phthisical patients.

3. Various headaches; periodic, esp. every seventh day; begin in occiput, spread upwards and settle over right eye; often end in vomiting; < at M.P. and **at climaxis**; sick headaches begin morning, increase during day and last till evening; > lying quiet in dark room; > sleep.

4. Naso-pharyngeal and ear complaints esp. with polypoid conditions.

5. Burning in various localities; hot palms and soles (Sulph.) climacteric flushes.

6. Pains in places where bones least covered, e.g. tibiæ, dorsi of hands, etc.

7. Lung complaints, even acute T.B. with hectic fever; **circumscribed redness of one or both cheeks**, sputa offensive even to patient.

8. Rheumatic pains in right arm and shoulder, < night in bed; cannot raise the arm.

9. Right-sided complaints.

10. **Modalities**; > lying quiet, in dark room.

SECALE CORNUTUM

1. Tall, thin, scrawny, feeble women of lax muscular fibre; old, decrepit subjects.

2. Extreme debility with restlessness, great anxiety and fear of death.

3. Collapse in choleroid and other diseases, hippocratic face with contortion esp. about the mouth; **skin cold to touch yet external warmth**, covering, etc., **intolerable.**

4. Passive hæmorrhages; blood copious, dark, think, watery, offensive; flow < motion.

5. Tendency to putrescence of all discharges.

6. Gangrenous conditions; of eruptions, etc.; dry, senile gangrene < external heat; small, painful boils with green contents.

7. Numbness and formication with or without paralysis; spastic paralysis.

8. Burning as of sparks falling on the parts.

9. Disorders of pregnancy and puerperium; labour pains prolonged, ineffectual or entirely wanting; **everything seems loose and open** but no expulsive power; (200th).

10. Patient chilly yet < external warmth; **markedly < covering up.**

SEPIA OFFICINALIS

1. Tall, slim (not conspicuously thin) women with narrow pelvices, dark hair, yellow complexion and characteristic "saddle"; "washerwoman's remedy".

2. Marked **indifference** even to family; no enjoyment in life; sits and says nothing; occasional fits of temper, then spiteful, obstinate and touchy. **Melancholy,** inspired by proud, stoical self-pity; < **consolation and company**; dreads meeting friends esp. men; **lachrymose,** weeps when detailing symptoms; anxiety and fear about real and imaginary evils so dreads being quite alone; disinclination to mental and physical labour.

3. Hypersensitiveness to external stimuli esp. noise and music; often causes the irritability.

4. Atony of digestive organs; **sinking feeling** at about 11 a.m. not > eating; nausea at the smell of food; hates fats, likes acids and pungent things; < milk; constipation from inactivity of rectum; with protruding piles.

5. Atony of female pelvic organs; irregular menses of nearly every form; **great pressure and bearing down,** must cross legs to prevent protrusion; char. h/a, extreme exhaustion and faintness in a.m. during M.P. Disorders during pregnancy and after.

6. Irregularities of circulation esp. at **climaxis**; e.g. flushes run upward and end in sweating and faintness; hands and feet hot alternately.

7. Micturition; frequent urging even at night; urine turbid, offensive, leaving adhesive red sediment; enuresis of children **during fist sleep**. Old gonorrhoeas.

8. Chronic skin conditions; yellow patches on face and body esp. chest and abdomen; chloasma; ringworm in isolated spots esp. on upper part of body; itching; esp. of genitalia, not > scratching. Easy sweating esp. between folds of skin; great **falling of hair**; warty growths.

9. Sensatin as of a ball in various organs (spasmodic contractions).

10. Lack of vital heat; **very chilly** yet < stuffy rooms; < **before thunder**; sultry, moist weather; < laundry work; many symptoms > violent exertion; < excitement.

Notes : Inimical to Lachesis mutus and Pulsatilla nigricans. A chronic of Nux vomica. A single dose often acts curatively for many weeks.

Keynote : **Atony.**

SILICEA TERRA

1. Subjects of light complexion and fine, dry skin; pale face, lax fibre; nervous, sanguine temperament; lacking in "grit". Specially suited to scrofulous, rachitic children with **large sweaty head and big abdomen; open fontanelles and sutures**; weak ankles, slow learning to walk, etc.

2. Patient anxious, yielding, timid (Puls.) but irritable if aroused; melancholy, lachrymose, desires consolation; lacks self-confidence but gets through by force of will. Children often obstinate and headstrong but cry when spoken to kindly (Iod.). Frightful dreams; somnambulism.

3. Hypersensitiveness, mental and physical, esp. to noise.

4. Chronic headaches, vertigo and cold sensations from **nape of neck to vertex**; headache from spine extending over head and locating over one eye esp. the right (Sang.); < draught, uncovering; > pressure, **wrapping up**, profuse urination, lying down in quiet, dark room.

5. Constipation from **paralytic weakness of rectum; stool partly expelled then recedes** (Thuj.); before and during menses; distension of abdomen with emission of offensive flatus; dislikes fat, < milk.

6. Unhealthy skin; every injury suppurates; indurations, scars and thickenings; malformation of nails; in-growing toe nails; promotes expulsion of foreign bodies from the tissues. Bad effects of vaccination (Thuj.).

7. **Suppurations** esp. long-lasting; of glands and joints; matures abscesses (low potencies) and heals after discharge; streptococcal infections; chronic ulceration fistulæ; whitlows.

8. **Offensive sweats** esp. of the **feet**; ailments from suppression of sweat or any discharges; feet and hands clammy.

9. Sticking, stitching, stabbing pains, gen, < motion.

10. **Lack of vital heat**; icy coldness of various parts; < **cold** esp. at approach of winter; < during new and waxing moon; all symptoms > warmth (except gastric); esp. > **wrapping up the head**; approach of summer, humid weather.

Notes : Incompatible with Mercury. Chronic of Pulsatilla nigricans. Slow but deep-acting remedy. Use cautiously in phthisical cases, avoiding high potencies.

STAPHYSAGRIA

1. Scrofulous or syphilitic subjects; elderly persons.

2. Mental hypersensitiveness; offended at trifles; continual concern about the future; peevishness, sometimes violent temper; children petulantly push or throw away things for which they cried; apathy, depression.

3. Ailments from mental emotions esp. pride, envy, chagrin, indignation, unmerited insults, etc.

4. Caries of the teeth; at edges; in scrofulous or syphilitic children; in women during pregnancy; toothache during M.P. < touch of food or drink, not on biting or chewing.

5. **Sexual disorders** with hypersensitiveness of generative organs; mental and physical effects of onanism and excesses; guilty, abashed look; mind persistently dwells on sexual subjects.

6. Prostatic troubles in old men; burning in urethra when not urinating; urging and pain after, in women, prolapse of uterus with relaxed, hanging-down feeling in abdomen, wants to support with hands; backache always < night in bed and in morning before rising.

7. **Injuries** from sharp cutting instruments, glass etc.; neuralgias after **surgical operations**.

8. Moist itching eruptions; after scratching, burning and itching appears elsewhere; figwarts, condylomata, etc.

9. Affections of the eyelids; **styes**, tumours, **nodosities**, chalazæ, etc.

10. **Modalities**; < cold; least **touch** affected parts; **mental emotions**; < **tobacco** esp. the cough.

Note : Inimical to Ran–b.

SULPHUR

1. Scrofulous, plethoric persons with very red lips; subject to skin eruptions esp. acne; hasty in temper and motion; often **untidy and dirty**-"ragged philosopher"-spare, stoop-shouldered, slack, shiftless, sensitive, sedentary. Emaciated children with big bellies, **intolerant of bathing and covering**; often dirty habits.

2. Mental and physical inertia; selfish, self-important, obstinate; chronic grumbler; melancholy yet often full of daydreams (even illusions) producing a foolish kind of happiness; lack of concentration; weak memory esp. for names and recent events; over sensitiveness to bad odours.

3. **Burnings everywhere** esp. vertex, palms and soles at night; puts feet out of bed; > cold.

4. All **discharges burning, excoriating** and generally offensive.

5. Local congestions esp. at **climaxis**; flashes of heat, faintness followed by sweating (Sep, Lach.); often assoc. with **sinking, all-gone sensation** in the fore-noon (Phos., Sep.).

6. Gastro-intestinal disorders; marked hunger and thirst yet stays thin; or drinks much, eats little; much flatulence with borborygmus and emissions of gas; < milk; liking for sweet things; usually constipation with piles; **stools large and painful** (makes child afraid to go to stool); acute attacks of **diarrhoea** esp. in the **morning**; urgent, **driving out of bed** (Aloe).

96

7. Skin dirty, diseased; every injury suppurates; **eruptions** of every kind esp. **pustular**; < warmth, esp. of bed at night washing; must scratch but leaves burning; boils in crops; chronic ailments with history of suppressed eruptions.

8. Catnap sleep; slightest noise awakens then difficulty in getting to sleep again; sleepy yet always wakes up unrefreshed.

9. **Complaints constantly relapsing**; also arouses **defective reaction** esp. in acute diseases; facilitates absorption of serous and inflammatory exudations; when paucity of symptoms often serves to bring out the true drug picture.

10. **Modalities**; < heat (except h/a) must have air yet may be sensitive to cold; < **warmth of bed**; slightest change of temperature esp. skin symptoms; midday and midnight; **standing still**; bathing.

Notes : Chronic of Aconitum napellus. Most used remedy in dark-skinned races. Prescribe with caution in phthisical patients. Sulphur and Lycopodium clavatum do not follow one another well; remember Sulph., Calc., Lyc. order.

SYPHILINUM

(Leuticum)

1. Subjects with **specific history** whose chancres have been treated by local means resulting in many years of suffering, esp. with skin and throat troubles; also congenital syphilis.

2. Weakness or loss of memory, esp. for names; feels as if going insane; terrible dread of the night owing to aggravation of all symptoms then; **despairs of recovery**.

3. In syphilitic affections when best selected remedy fails to relieve or permanently improve.

4. **Great falling of the hair.**

5. Pains increase and decrease gradually; shift locality; < **night.**

6. **Craving for alcohol** in any form; hereditary tendency to alcoholism; constipation the rule.

7. Eruptions of the skin; dull red, copper-coloured spots becoming blue when patient is cold.

8. **Leucorrhoea; profuse, soaks through napkin** and runs down to the heels (Alum).

9. Rheumatic complaints esp. of shoulder or at insertion of deltoid, < raising arm laterally.

10. **Modality**; always < **twilight to daylight** (rev. Med.).

THUJA OCCIDENTALIS

1. Fleshy persons; dark, shiny, greasy complexion esp. forehead; black hair and unhealthy skin; lymphatic temperament. Hydrogenoid constitution.

2. Depression even to melancholia; dislikes company; weary of life, peevish, quarrelsome; loss of memory; excitable, always in a hurry. **Fantastic fixed ideas**: (a) of strange person by his side, (b) of separation of soul and body, (c) of animal or something alive in the abdomen, (d) of brittleness, as if body and limbs made of glass, (e) of domination by some superior power.

3. **Sycosis** and **vaccinosis**; ailments from vaccination (esp. diarrhoea), suppressed gonorrhoeas (esp. rheumatic arthritis) and chronic effects of tea-drinking, meat-eating and smoking.

4. Chronic headaches with mental confusion; pain dull or as if pierced by a nail (Coff., Ign.); < morning on waking or evening at bedtime, preventing sleep; > open air. Vertigo on closing the eyes (Lach., Ther.).

5. Chronic muco-purulent discharges; green, sanious, offensive; often with ulceration of mucous membrane.

6. Alimentary disorders; (a) pyorrhoea with caries of teeth; roots decay, crowns relatively sound; (b) constipation, **stool recedes** after partial expulsion; large, hard, black balls; with piles, pain < when sitting; fissures at anus, etc.; (c) diarrhoea, **sudden**, copious, explosive **gurgling**; < early a.m.

7. **Overgrowths of mucous and cutaneous tissue;** papillomata, fibromata, condylomata, figwarts, polypi, etc., soft, humid with unpleasant secretion, bleed easily; also styes, tarsal tumours, etc.

8. Skin, looks dirty; nails deformed, brittle; hair falls out or splits; eruptions only on covered parts. **Sweats only on uncovered parts** or all over except head (rev. Sil.); while asleep, stops on waking (rev. Samb.); sweats at all the orifices (Nit.–ac.). pustular eruptions.

9. Left-sided ovaritis esp. chronic; < during M.P., must lie down; periods usually premature, scanty.

10. **Modalities;** < damp, esp. cold, damp air, bathing, etc.; heat of bed; sometimes prefers cold to heat; < **morning** and continues throughout the day; or or after 3 a.m.; narcotics.

Note : Use with care during pregnancy as it tends to produce abortion.

TUBERCULINUM

(Bacillinum)

1. Fair, blue-eyed subjects. Tall, slim, flat-chested; blue sclerotic, red lips; mentally precocious but physically weak; child often covered with fine hairs on chest, back, etc. **Tubercular diathesis.**

2. Despondency with irritability; taciturn, sulky; disposition naturally sweet but changed by disease; desires constant change; **fears dogs.**

3. **Symptoms ever changing** locality; begin suddenly and cease suddenly.

4. **Always catching cold** without knowing how or where .

5. **Emaciation rapid** and pronounced; often in spite of good appetite; patient easily tires.

6. Chronic tubercular headaches, from above right eye to occiput; h/a of school-girls < slightest mental exertion; glasses fail to >.

7. Chronic diarrhoea with great weakness and profuse night sweat; esp. in early a.m., sudden and imperative (Sulph).

8. Chronic dysmenorrhoeas; periods premature, profuse, protracted.

9. Skin complaints; tubercular **eczemas** over entire body, intense itching < undressing, bathing, oozing in folds of

skin and in the hair with rawness and soreness; immense quantities of white, bran-like scales. Crops of very painful small boils appear successively in the nose with green, foetid pus. **Ringworm.**

10. Patient < **heat**, yet sensitive to cold; exertion.

Note : Valuable when well-selected remedies fail in patients with family history of T.B.

VERATRUM ALBUM

1. Thin, choleric, emotional subjects deficient in vital reaction; extremes of life and young people of nervous, sanguine temperament.

2. Violent manias, deliriums, with anger and rage; habits dirty and destructive esp. to clothes; attacks often alt. sullen silence; may be religious excitement.

3. **Sudden collapse with cold sweat** esp. on forehead; hippocratic features, etc.; coldness and blueness of body surface yet covering does not > but rather <.

4. Acute, **violent vomiting and purging**; stools gen. watery, greenish, flaky; with cramps and cutting colic; in choleraic diseases; from cold; from fruit, vegetables; esp. suddenly at night in summer. More chronic states have constipation with much straining.

5. **All discharges are copious** (vomit, urine, motions, sweat, etc.).

6. Intense thirst with desire for large quantities of cold drinks.

7. **Local frigidities**; icy coldness of vertex, etc., yet often sense of internal burning.

8. Neuralgias, headaches and dysmenorrhoeas with prostration, even vomiting and cold sweat; < heat; pain compels patient to walk about yet no >. Dysmenorrhoea with violent emotional disturbances. Rheumatic pains < during wet weather; warmth of bed.

9. Cardiac troubles after severe or prolonged illness; pulse slow and weak, thready; blood pressure low (cases where Crataegus oxyacantha so often valuable); frequent faintings; red face turns pale on sitting up suddenly.

10. **Modalities**; < night; motion; drinking; before and during discharges; after fright.

Keynote : **Violence.**

VERATRUM VIRIDE

1. Plethoric subjects.

2. Furious deliriums; screaming and howling.

3. Sudden, intense local congestions esp. to base of brain, spine, chest, stomach; also of pelvis, dysmenorrhoea (Caul.); coup-de-soleil.

4. Acute febrile diseases with great arterial excitement; convulsions often precede eruptions; acute rheumatis.

5. Tongue white or yellow-coated with **red streak down center.**

6. **Slow pulse** is primary and more characteristic action (Dig.); arterial excitement is secondary effect.

7. Convulsive twitchings and tremblings, even paralysis with tingling.

8. Cerebro-spinal diseases with cold, clammy perspiration, opisthotonos; **basilar meningitis**; apoplexy with slow, full, hard-as-iron pulse.

9. **Pneumonias**; early congestive stage with slow, laboured breathing and livid face (mother tincture or low potency).

10. **Modalities**;< on rising, waking, evening, motion.

ZINCUM METALLICUM

1. Cachectic, emaciated persons whose constitutions have broken down through stress of life; **vitality deficient,** circulation poor; nervous exhaustion from overwork.

2. Soporous conditions of the mind; child repeats everything said to it.

3. Hypersensitiveness to external stimuli.

4. General trembling assoc. with chronic disease; weakness and trembling of extremities esp. lower limbs; **legs or feet extremely fidgety** (of hands-kali–br.); varicose conditions (Puls.).

5. Incipient brain troubles esp. from suppressed eruptions; sudden alarming symptoms follow disappearances of erupation.

6. **Discharges** and eruptions difficult owing to weakness of patient but they **always** > ; menstrual flow > all her symptoms (e.g. neuralgia of left ovary).

7. Convulsions with pale face; no heat (ctr. Bell.); automatic muscular movements; twitchings and jerkings esp. during sleep at night; child rolls head from side to side.

8. **Spinal affections** with burning whole length of spine; also dull backache much < sitting.

9. **Ravenous hunger esp. at 11 a.m.**; sinking sensation (Sulph.); great greediness when eating.

10. **Modalities**; < cold; evenings; mental and physical exertion; wine and other strong stimulants (and knows it); milk; sugar; > camphor.

Notes : Inimical to Cham., Nux–v. Sometimes chronic of Ignatia amara.

AESCULUS HIPPOCASTANUM

1. **Fullness** in various parts; venous congestions.

2. Irritability, feels and is miserably cross.

3. Mucous membranes dry, swollen, burning, feel raw; sometimes thin, watery, acrid dischages; mouth, throat and rectum particularly affected.

4. Rectal disorders with char. fullness, burning and dryness, **rectum feels as if full of sticks or splinters**; intense pain at anus for hours after stool; constipation with haemorrhoids which are usually blind, very sensitive; prolapsus ani.

5. **Severe dull backache in sacro-lumbar region with lame feeling**; fullness and distress in liver region; pain < walking, stooping forward.

ALOE SOCOTRINA

1. Phlegmatic, indolent persons; old people; women near climaxis; tendency to local congestions.

2. Periodic and alternating complaints; e.g. congestive h/a in winter, diarrhoea in summer.

3. Diarrhoea spluttery, immediately after eating and drinking (Crot-t.); **drives out of bed early a.m.** (Sulph.); abdominal distension with rumbling and **colic** before and during stool > passing flatus and stool but prostration and sweating.

4. Constipation, solid stool passes without exertion or unnoticed; passage of **mucus in jelly-like lumps. Haemorrhoids** protrude like bunch of grapes after each stool with bleeding, bearing down, itching, burning, > cold applications.

5. **Modalities**; < hot, dry weather; walking and standing, > open air; cool applications.

BENZOICUM ACIDUM

1. Uric acid diathesis esp. if gonorrheal or syphilitic taint.

2. **Urine dark, brownish with intensely strong, odour** in urinary or other complaints.

3. Rheumatic and arthritic conditions; gouty concretions; tearing stitching joint pains < cold open air,> wrapping up; ganglia.

4. Diarrhoea in children; profuse, watery, very offensive, exhausting stools of urinous odour; characteristic urine.

5. Symptoms tend to travel from left to right and from below upward.

BERBERIS VULGARIS

1. Complaints with renal or vesical symptoms predomidating; esp. rheumatic and arthiritic affections.

2. Renal colic; with passage of calculi; stitching, **cutting pains in kidney region following course of ureter into Bladder and urethra**; esp. left side.

3. Bilious and gastro-intestinal disorders, esp. hepatic colic from passage of gall-stones; with jaundice.

4. Backache with stiffness, lameness and numbness,< touch, pressure, sitting, stooping, lying, > standing still; burning and soreness in kidney region.

5. **Modalities**; < motion, esp. sudden jarring; > open air.

BISMUTHUM

1. **Great restlessness with anguish** (Ars.); cannot keep still; sits then walks, then lies down, never long in one place.

2. **Solitude unbearable**; craves company; child wants to hold mother's hand continually.

3. Gastric disorder esp. gastralgia; pain severe, burning, pressive, extending to spine; **vomiting; of water as soon as it reaches stomach**, in enormous quantities; with convulsive gagging and inexpressible pain; after laparotomy, etc.

4. Bowel complaints with loose, offensive, debilitating stools; when vomiting predominates.

5. Alternating symptoms and complaints; e.g. headache and gastralgia.

BROMIUM

1. Acts best in persons with light-blue eyes, flaxen hair, fair skin; **blonde**, red-cheeked, scrofulous girls (ctr. Iod.).

2. Inflammatory diseases of respiratory tract esp. upper part; **croupous conditions** with much rattling of mucus during cough; severe suffocative attack; spasmodic constriction of larynx; hoarseness; chest pains running upwards; also obstinate coryzas.

3. Swelling and induration of glands esp. in scrofulous children.

4. Diphtheria when membrane invades larynx; extending upwards.

5. **Modalities**; < evening to midnight; warm room; left side;> at the seaside (Iod).

CACTUS GRANDIFLORUS

1. **Fear of death** (more persistent than in Acon.) esp. in plethoric persons subject to lacal congestions.

2. **Constrictive sensation** as of hoop in various organs; **of whole body** as if caged, each wire being twisted lighter and tighter; with numbness.

3. **Cardiac troubles**, acute and chronic, with char. constriction; heart feels as if rapidy clasped and unclasped by an iron hand, preventing normal movement; oppression of breathing.

4. Haemorrhages; from nose, lungs, stomach, uterus, bladder, etc.

5. Intermittent fevers with regular periodicity, esp. every day at the same hour; with anguish, oppressed breathing, etc.

CALENDULA OFFICINALIS

1. **Wounds** of all kinds esp. cuts or lacerations of soft parts: with or without loss of substance; promotes healthy granulation and prevents excessive suppuration; after surgical operations.

2. Old, neglected, offensive wounds, threatening gangrene; much sloughing of soft parts.

3. Rupture of muscles or tendons, with much soreness and pain; compound fractures.

4. Ulcers of various kinds with excessive discharge of pus; painful as if beaten.

5. Exhaustion from loss of blood and excessive pain.

Note : Use locally and internally. Locally the Succus is the best preparation.

CAPSICUM ANNUUM

1. Fair persons of plethoric habit; phlegmatic, indolent, dread cold, open air, exercise, and society; clumsy. Fat, dirty children.

2. **Burning, smarting pains** and sensation not > by heat; esp. of mucous membranes; associated with **constriction and chilliness.**

3. Throat conditions < when not swallowing (lgn.) esp. in smokers and alcoholics.

4. Chronic suppuration of the ear; mastoid involved; swelling behind ear, painful, extremely sore and sensitive to touch.

5. Threatened gangrene of lung; each explosive cough expelling a pungent, foetid odour; pain in distant parts on coughing, esp. head.

CARBO ANIMALIS

1. Diseases of elderly persons with marked **venous plethora**; feeble circulation, no vital heat; want of energy; dislikes conversation and company.

2. **Glands, indurated**, swollen, even ulcerated; with lancinating, burning pains; tendency to malignancy; scirrhus, bluish appearance, esp. axillary, mammary and inguinal glands.

3. **Discharges** gen. offensive and **always exhausting**; e.g. during menstruation so weak can hardly speak.

4. Joints and muscles weak; sprains and strains on slight exertion.

5. **Modalities**; < open, dry, cold air, after shaving (ctr. Brom.).

CAULOPHYLLUM THALICTROIDES

1. Chilly, nervous women esp. if with " moth patches" on forehead (Sep.).

2. Internal trembling.

3. Spasmodic disorders of female system; **dysmenorrhoea** with irregular spasmodic pains and bearing down esp. left ovarian region (almost specific, cp. Mag–p., Vib.). **In labour** with rigid os. **Pains spasmodic irregular and ineffectual**, nervous excitement; after-pains. Leucorrhoea acrid, exhausting; in little girls.

4. Nervous, spasmodic complaints during the establishment or the menstrual function.

5. Rheumatism of small joints esp. wrists and fingers; pains intermittent, erratic, change place every few minutes (Puls.).

Note : Strongly antidoted by coffee.

CICUTA VIROSA

1. Spasmodic affections esp. **convulsions** with loss of consciousness; pulis dilated, insensible; **frightful contortions of limbs** and whole body; opisthotonos; frothing at mouth, etc; spasms renewed by touch, noise, jarring; followed by great exhaustion; from indigestion, dentition, worms, repercussed eruptions, etc.; epilepsies, choreas.

2. Abnormal appetite for indigestible things.

3. Chronic effects of concussion of brain or spine, esp. spasms.

4. Vesicular and pustular eruptions with formation of yellowish honey-coloured crusts, esp. about corners of mouth; little or no itching.

5. Violent shocks in various localities causing jerking of the part; sudden detonations in the ears on swallowing esp. in deafness of old people.

CINA MARITIMA

1. Children (esp. dark-haired) with **worm affections**; pale face, white about the mouth, boring of nose with finger, grinding of teeth at night, restless sleep, hunger, fever, etc.

2. **Ill-humour**; cannot be quieted; dislikes caresses; rejects everything offered; may want to be carried but is no better.

3. Spasmodic affections esp. convulsions, chorea, whooping cough; from intestinal irritation, particularly worms.

4. **Ravenous appetite**; hunger soon after full meal; craves many and different things, sweets.

5. Fevers, remittent, stimulating worm fever; intermittent, in children, daily attacks at same hour; no thirst during chill or heat.

Note : The alkaloid **Santoninum** is specific for Ascaris Lumbricodes.

COLOCYNTHIS

1. Extreme **irritability** and impatience esp. in rheumatic subjects; ailments from mental emotions esp. anger with indignation.

2. **Severe colic** > **bending double** (rev. Diosc.) **or hard pressure**; patient presses hard things against abdomen> stool or passage of flatus; < cheese; < 4-9 p.m.

3. Neuralgias esp. of larger nerves < touch yet > hard pressure, rest and warmth; particularly right-sided sciatica and ovaralgia; vomiting and diarrhoea often result from the pain.

4. Diarrhoea and dysentery brought on by chill during hot weather, < eating and drinking; with char. colic, > stool.

5. Vertigo esp. on turning head to the left.

CROCUS SATIVUS

1. Rapid alternation of mental states; **true hysteria**; sudden change from greatest hilarity to deepest gloom; extremely happy, affectionate, wants to kiss everybody, next moment in a rage.

2. **Haemorrhages** from any part; blood **dark, clotted forming long black streams from bleeding surface**; < slightest motion; esp. epistaxis and metrorrhagia.

3. Sensation as of something alive moving about in various organs; in hysterical states; imaginary pregnancy (Thuj).

4. Spasmodic contractions and twitching of single muscles; of the lids in eye disease; chorea.

5. **Modalities**; >open air; headache < during menstrul flow.

CROTALUS HORRIDUS

1. Adynamic conditions in general, esp. **low, malignant fevers**; great prostration, low muttering delirium, tongue dry, brown, cracked or yellow with brown center and red edges, etc. Bubonic and pneumonic plague.

2. Haemorrhagic tendencies; from any or all orifices, from gums, under skin, nails, etc.

3. **Septicaemia states**; zymotic or septic poisonings; prolonged suppurations; gangrenous tendencies, discharges putrid; septic conditions of abdomen when pus retained.

4. Yellow skin and conjunctivae, malignant jaundice; **yellow fever.**

5. General symptoms and modalities similar to Lachesis mutus.

DIGITALIS PURPUREA

1. **Cardiac diseases** with great anxiety; dyspnoea, sudden sensation as if heart stood still; **pulse** feeble, irregular, fluttering, **intermittent or extremely slow**; any motion esp. rising from bed or chair causes rapid, weak, jerky pulse and sometimes cyanosis, even syncope.

2. Patient low-spirited, tearful; likes consolation; anxiety even apart from heart disease.

3. **Dropsies**; all forms of cardiac origin.

4. Liver disorders with enlargement and induration; jaundice; urine scanty, high-coloured; stools ashy-white; soreness in liver region.

5. Seminal weakness with weak heart; involuntary emissions at night with or without dreams; also acute prostatic troubles.

DROSERA ROTUNDIFOLIA

1. Spasmodic catarrhal affections of respiratory tract; esp. **whooping cough**; violent paroxysms follow one another so rapidly that child cannot get breath; often ends in gagging, vomiting and cold sweat; sometimes with hemorrhage from nose or mouth.

2. **Coughs** in general < **lying down and after midnight**, warmth, drinking, using voice, etc.; patient badly shaken up, must hold sides; coughs gen. end with free discharge of mucus.

3. Constant titillating cough beginning as soon as head touches pillow at night; esp. in children.

4. Valuable in **tubercular diseases**; phthisis, esp. laryngeal cases; T.B. of long bones.

5. Measles with hoarse, spasmodic cough.

DULCAMARA

1. Phlegmatic scrofulous subjects with low vitality. Children who dislike sweats.

2. Vrious complaints (catarrhal, rheumatic, dropsical, etc.) from exposure to or < **by damp, cold atmosphere** (Lemm., Nat–s.) esp. sudden changes in hot weather (Bry.), < evening and night.

3. Suppression of discharges or retrocession of eruptions from damp air, working in water.

4. Delicate skin esp. liable to nettlerash over whole body, often precedes M.P.; chronic vesicular eruptions even to ulceration; large, smooth fleshy warts.

5. Paralysis of single parts; parts feel cold.

EUPATORIUM PERFOLIATUM

1. Worn-out constitutions; from inebriety; from bilious or intermittent fevers.

2. Diseases characterized by **intense aching pains in bones** as if broken, and bruised feeling all over the body surface.

3. Intermittent fevers; bone pains before and during chill; violent headache; **vomiting**, from drink of water, **of bile as chill passes off**; thirst begins several hours before chill, continues during chill and heat; sweating stage almost or entirely wanting.

4. **Influenzas** with symptoms as (2); painful soreness in eyeballs, much sneezing, hacking cough; prostration, etc.

5. Pains come suddenly and go suddenly.

EUPHRASIA OFFICINALIS

1. Acute catarrhal affections esp. of eyes and nose; **profuse acrid lachrymation with profuse bland coryza** (rev. All-c.); often assoc. soreness and pressive pain behind sternum and hacking cough with free mucous expectoration; cough only during daytime, < on rising a.m.; influenza; whooping cough.

2. Conjunctivitis; acute with excessive, acrid watery discharge; sub-acute with profuse, mattery discharge making cheeks sore; accumulation of mucus on cornea causing frequent blinking to effect removal; photophobia; lid margins swollen, red, burning, even ulcerating.

3. Menstrual disorders; **flow lasts only one hour** or late and lasting only one day.

4. Ailments resulting from falls; contusions, or mechanical injuries to external parts.

5. **Modalities**; < evening or on rising a.m.; indoors; warmth; south winds; > outdoors.

FERRUM PHOSPHORICUM

1. **First stage of inflammatory diseases** before exudation takes place; heat with soft, full quick pulse (lacks Acon. tension); thirst; sweating does not > pains; in mucous inflammations discharge gen. blood-streaked.

2. Complaints from taking cold or suppressed perspiration esp. inflammation of mucous tracts; special affinity for lungs and stomach.

3. Tendency to sudden local congestions, esp. in pale anaemic persons.

4. Hemorrhages; bright blood from any outlet.

5. Articular rheumatism with fever, shooting pains < movements yet sometimes > gentle motion; < 4-6 a.m and p.m.

FLUORICUM ACIDUM

1. Complaints of old age or prematurely old-looking persons, even children; broken-down constitutions esp. from abuse of alcohol or from mercurio-syphilitic dyscrasia.

2. Disposition to constant and rapid motion; "seems as if she could walk for ever"

3. **Bone diseases** esp. long bones; caries with thin, excoriating discharge; of mastoid process; bone fistulae esp. dental and lachrymal.

4. Varicose veins and ulcers; bedsores; naevi; old cicatrices which become red. Itching, and threatening ulceration.

5. General resemblance to Silicea Terra but modality reversed < heat, > cold.

GLONOINUM

1. **Cerebral congestions** esp. **from exposure to sun** or radiated heat; from mental excitement; at climaxis; face may be pale or congested even to dusky appearance. **Sunstroke**.

2. Mental confusion; familiar things seem strange; loses his way; after injuries, etc.

3. **Throbbing pulsation all through head with every pulse beat; not painful.**

4. Headaches; severe bursting or crushing pain, < noise, motion, jarring, stooping, touch of hat, having hair cut; sudden attacks; from heat of sun; in place of menses.

5. Congestion of heart; often alt. rush of blood to head; angina pectoris with fluttering of heart and violent beating as if chest would burst open, laboured breathing; pains radiate in all directions even into arms (3x).

HAMAMELIS VIRGINIANA

1. **Venous congestions**; varicose veins and ulcers, phlebitis; ecchymoses; heamorrhoids bluish, bleeding, gen. without constipation.

2. **Venous haemorrhages** from any orifice; flow dark gen. profuse.

3. Bruised soreness of affected parts; even in rheumatism.

4. Wounds, esp. incised or ragged; relieves the pain and soreness.

5. **Modalities**; < open air, esp. moist warm air; motion; at M.P.

HELLEBORUS NIGER

1. Weakly, scrofulous children prone to brain troubles. esp. at dentition.

2. Melancholia; silent despair; stupidity or unintelligent muttering; < consolation; irritability; mind loses control over body, strong concentration needed before muscles will act.

3. **Acute brain affections**; hydrocephalus, during stage of effusion; stupefaction or insensibility; **head rolls from side to side, bores into pillow** or is beaten with hands; sudden screams; eyes wide open, pupils insensible to light; chewing motions with mouth; grinding of teeth; automatic motion of one arm or leg; urine gen. suppressed; may be convulsions. Meningitis.

4. **Sudden dropsical swellings**; urine red or black scanty; coffee-ground sediment; or urine suppressed; char. stupefaction and mental torpor.

5. **Modalities**; < 4-9 p.m. (Lyc.) esp. sinking sensation and h/a.

HYOSCYAMUS NIGER

1. **Acute mania**; patient, talkative, quarrelsome, gen. **lascivious**, exposes the person, etc.; in the between state, **suspicious** depression; fears solitude, poison, plots. Ailments from jealousy, unfortunate love, mental emotions.

2. **Delirium** during course of acute diseases; temperature not markedly high; restless, picks bedclothes, etc.; beclouded senses; staring eyes; dry tongue, etc.; involuntary urine and faeces; stands midway between Bell. and Stram. lacking cerebral congestion of former and fierce, raging mania of latter. Delirium tremens.

3. Spasmodic affections without consciousness; every muscle twitches from eye to toes; opisthotonos; **convulsions**, of children from fright, worms; of pregnant or parturient women.

4. Nervous coughs; teasing, dry, spasmodic, < on lying down, > sitting up (Dros.); < night, using voice, eating, drinking.

5. Insomnia in irritable, excitable subjects; from business difficulties or other nervous excitement; drowsy yet restless; in children, with twitchings and startings from fright.

HYPERICUM PERFORATUM

1. Bad effects of **brain or spinal concussion**; esp. headache with sensation as if being lifted up high into air.

2. Punctured, incised or lacerated **wounds, esp. of parts rich in sentient nerves** as fingers, toes, matrices of nails; intense pain and soreness; injuries from treading on nails, splinters, etc.; prevents tetanus; useful after amputations.

3. Spinal affections, traumatic or otherwise, with extreme sensitiveness of cervical vertebrae to touch, patient screams if approached; slightest motion of neck or arm extorts cries.

4. Consequences of shock or fright; **shell shock**; neurasthenia after injuries or surgical operations.

5. Neuralgias, esp. when no other remedy seems specially indicated; parts excessively painful and sore; < change of weather. **Neuritis.**

KALIUM BROMATUM

1. Large, fleshy people; particularly children and young persons. Patients suffering from **brain fag** with numb feeling in head as if would lose reason; **loss of memory,** forgets how to talk; fits of uncontrollable weeping and profound melancholic delusions, even mania.

2. Nervous restlessness, must keep busy; **fidgety hands** (feet-Zinc.); restless and sleeplessness at night, from worry, etc.; somnambulism.

3. Spasms-inco-ordination of muscles-paralysis, stammering speech; staggering gait; epileptiform convulsions, etc.

4. **Anaesthesia** of various parts or of entire body; esp. of fauces from alcoholism.

5. **Acne-like eruptions** esp. on face, chest and shoulders (Eug.).

KALMIA LATIFOLIA

1. Acute, sub-acute and chronic **rheumatism**; pains severe, suddenly change locality, going from joint to joint, with numbness, gen. < early part of night or soon after going to bed.

2. **Cardiac diseases** assoc. with rheumatism or in post-influenzal conditions; violent shooting, stabbing pains; palpitation; great dyspnoea; slow, weak pulse; gen. pale face, anxious expression, cold extremities; < lying left side.

3. **Neuralgias** attended or succeeded **by numbness of the parts; pains shoot in a downward direction**; lightning pains of table dorsalis.

4. Deep-seated eye affections with sense of stiffness around eyes and in eyelids; severe stitching pains < turning eyes, begin at sunrise and last till noon, or < at noon, leave at sunset (Nat-m.); h/a with similar modalities.

5. Symptoms predominantly right-sided.

MAGNESIUM PHOSPHORICUM

1. Tired, languid, worn-out subjects, esp. dark-complexioned, emaciated persons of highly nervous organization.

2. **Neuralgic pains, darting, lightnig-like in character**, > **warm applications, pressure, friction**; < touch, cold air, cold water, uncovering; paroxysmal pains of all kinds except burning.

3. Complaints purely spasmodic in character; no fever; etc.; in teething children; **cramps**, convulsions, choreas, coughs.

4. **Colic**; flatulent, forcing patient to bend double (Coloc.) > rubbing, warmth, pressure; belching gives no >. Menstrual colic with char. symptoms. > when flow begins. (Give in hot water.).

5. **Right side** of body mostly affected.

MERCURIUS CORROSIVUS

1. Invaluable in **violent, acute destructive inflammations** (phagedenic tendencies) of any part, esp. of mucous membranes; catarrhal, scrofulous, gonorrheal syphilitic.

2. Typical **dysentery**; scanty stools of pure mucus tinged or streaked with blood, colicky pains extreme, persistent **tenesmus** and burning; often acc. by tenesmus of bladder; no > stool.

3. Acute Inflammatory conditions of eyes and lids with swelling, intense pain, photophobia and acrid lachrymation.

4. Violent inflammation of serous membranes esp. peritoneum; peritonitis, **appendicitis,** etc., when abscess is about to form.

5. Acute or **chronic interstitial nephritis** with violent cystic symptoms; also gonorrhoeas with thick, greenish discharge.

Note : General symptoms and modalities as Merc.

MURIATICUM ACIDUM

1. Low, adynamic fevers; **typhoid states** with great debility, involuntary discharges, **lower jaw hangs down, slides down in bed**, sordes on teeth, tongue dry, shrunken, leather-like paralyzed; pulse feeble, breath offensive.

2. **Ulcerations** of gastrointestinal mucous membranes with greyish-white deposits; ulcers extremely sensitive to touch, deep, perforating, bluish or black base, bleed easily, tend to slough. Diphtheria; epithelioma.

3. Haemorrhoids; swollen, blue or dark purle, sensitive to touch; appear suddenly in children; in pregnant women; prolapsus ani.

4. **Involuntary stool while urinating; on passing flatus** (Aloe): from paralysis of sphincter ani.

5. Discharges thin, excoriating, putrid, debilitating, even from ulcers.

PYROGENIUM

1. **Sapraemic and septicemia conditions** when best selected remedy fails to relieve or permanently improve; onset of septic fevers with chill beginning in back, or general chill; **pulse very rapid**, small, wiry; may be out of all proportion to temperature; distinct consciousness of a heart.

2. **Bed feels hard;** parts lain on feel sore and bruised, causing great **restlessness**.

3. All excretions horribly offensive.

4. **Tongue**, large flabby, **fiery-red, clean, smooth as if varnished**; states sweetish, very foitid.

5. Constipation with complete inertia; obstinate from impaction; in fevers; **stool large, black, carrion-like** or small, black balls.

RANUNCULUS BULBOSUS

1. Neuralgic, myalgic or rheumatic pains; stitching, shooting esp. in **chest walls**; < damp weather, atmospheric changes.

2. **Intercostal rheumatism**; chest sore, bruised < touch, motion, turning body; pleurodynia.

3. Herpes zoster; dark-bluish transparent vesicles; preceded or followed by the characteristic neuralgic pains.

4. Hay fever; smarting, burning and tingling in eyes and nose; nostrils dry, obstructed. < evenings.

5. Bad effects of alcoholic liquors; delirium tremens.

RUTA GRAVEOLENS

1. **Mechanical injuries of bones** and periosteum; spirans, dislocations, with bruised pains; lameness after sprains esp. of wrists and ankles; **ganglia**; flat foot.

2. Bruised, lame sensation all over, < limbs and joints; parts lain on are painful as if bruised; even in rheumatic complaints.

3. Ailments from **overstraining the eyes**; headaches asthenopia, etc.; eyes burn and ache, feel strained or hot, like balls of fire.

4. Dyspepsia; after abdominal strain; when meat always disagrees, causing much distress and urticaria; also < milk.

5. Rectal complaints; **prolapse** immediately on attempting defecation; after confinement or undue strain; carcinoma of rectum.

SPIGELIA ANTHELMIA

1. Light-haired, anaemic, debilitated subjects of rheumatic diathesis; scrofulous children with worm troubles, esp. when stammering results; fear of sharp pointed things.

2. **Violent neuralgic pains**, chiefly left-sided, beginning one point and radiating all directions; from sunrise increasing till noon, then declining till sunset; **fifth pair nerves** specially involved; eye on affected side often waters; right sided ciliary neuralgia; **periodic headache** beginning base of brain or occiput, extending over head, settling over or about left eye (right-Sang., Sil.), < stooping.

3. Deep-seated eye troubles; even glaucoma; intense pressive pain, esp. on turning the eyes, as if too large for orbits.

4. **Organic heart affections** with violent, visible, audible palpitation; great dyspnoea, must lie on right side or with head high; purring feeling over heart, wave-like motion not sychoronous with pulse; systolic blowing at apex; pain goes down left arm; tobacco heart.

5. **Modalities**; < cold, damp, stormy weather; **noise, least jar, shake or movement**; body painfully sensitive to touch; toothache < smoking.

SPONGIA TOSTA

1. Fair-complexioned women and children of lax fibre timid and sensitive; tubercular diathesis.

2. Marked **anxiety**, even terror, in nearly all complaints; gen. assoc. with the **suffocative attacks**.

3. Great dryness of mucous membranes in respiratory tract **cough** with no mucous rale, dry, **sibilant, "like a saw through pine-board"** ; < sweets, cold drinks, lying with head low, sleep, mental excitement. **Croup**; after exposure to dry, cold winds; **anxious wheezing** < during inspiration: dry, barking cough in suffocative attacks; (often after Aconite has controlled the high fever and dry, hot skin); < after midnight.

4. **Heart diseases**; organic; suffocating attacks on lying flat with head low, esp. after midnight; hypertrophied conditions, esp. when assoc. emphysema; sudden failing of compensation; violent palpiatation; pain down left arm; < sleep.

5. Glandular enlargements; with induration; of thyroid (**goiter**), of generative organs, of testicles after suppressed gonorrhoea or maltreated orchitis.

STANNUM METALLICUM

1. Pale, anaemic subjects who suffer from dyspnoea and depression; feel like weeping all the time but weeping <. Children with worm troubles.

2. Great nervous and muscular prostration; so weak she drops into a chair; **weakness** (emptiness) is esp. **referred to the chest** (Arg–met.), < using the voice; often acc. by profuse, debilitating sweats with musty obour.

3. Neuralgic pains; gradually increase to a high degree then gradually decline (Plat.).

4. Chronic catarrhal troubles; sputa profuse, easily detached, light yellow, lumpy, tasting sweetish, salty or putrid (Stann–i. 3x).

5. **Modalities**; < cold; using voice; descending; warm drinks; > pressure.

STRAMONIUM

1. Young plethoric persons who desire light and company, **dread the dark and solitude.**

2. **Acute manias and deliriums**, great terror, attempts to escape, hallucinations esp. of terrible animals; great rage with screaming, biting and scratching; **loquacity, constant praying and entreating**; staring, brilliant eyes, widely dilated pupils; strange imaginations, e.g. of double personality, of scattered limbs, etc.

3. **Spasmodic complaints**; convulsions, chorea (facial muscles chiefly affected), epilepsies; from fright, renewed by bright light, sight of brilliant objects, attempts to swallow liquids; strabismus, stammering, **hydrophobia**.

4. **Painlessness** with most complaints > intense pain of suppuration particularly in abscess of left hip joint or in panaritum.

5. In fevers with intense, bright scarlet-red rash over whole body, and often suppression of all secretions and excretions.